WORKING WITH
DYSARTHRICS
A PRACTICAL GUIDE TO
THERAPY FOR DYSARTHRIA

WORKING WITH DYSARTHRICS

A PRACTICAL GUIDE TO THERAPY FOR DYSARTHRIA

SANDRA J ROBERTSON & FAY THOMSON

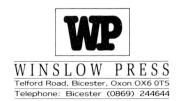

WINSLOW PRESS

Telford Road, Bicester, Oxon OX6 0TS
Telephone: Bicester (0869) 244644

First published in 1986 by Winslow Press,
Telford Road, Bicester, Oxon OX6 0TS
Reprinted 1987, 1989

ISBN 0 86388 034 7

02-100/Printed in Great Britain by
Hobbs the Printers, Southampton

CONTENTS

Sandra Robertson MSc, LCST, LLCM

Sandra Robertson has been principal lecturer and course director of the BSc Speech Pathology and Therapy course at Manchester Polytechnic since 1983.

After qualifying as a speech therapist from Jordanhill College of Education, Glasgow, she worked for several years in a number of Glasgow hospitals, including the Institute of Neurology and Neurosurgery at Killearn and the Southern General Hospital.

In 1971 she moved to London to take up a lecturing post at the former West End Hospital Speech Therapy Training School, now the National Hospitals College of Speech Sciences. After five years of lecturing, she returned to full-time hospital work as the Chief Speech Therapist for Harrow District Hospitals, based at Northwick Park Hospital. In 1978 she returned to the National Hospitals College of Speech Sciences to lecture and to help develop the BSc in Speech Sciences degree in conjunction with University College, London.

In 1977 she completed an MSc degree in Human Communications, which included research into the long-term effects of anti-epileptic drugs on speech. Her interest in acquired dysarthria has dominated her lecturing, research and clinical activities for a number of years and she has developed and published the Dysarthria Profile.

Sandra Robertson and Fay Thomson carried out a joint research project in 1982/3 in which they investigated the efficacy of intensive therapy and its long-term effects upon the performance of patients with Parkinson's disease.

Fay Thomson (YOUNG) MA, LCST

Fay Thomson qualified in London in 1974 and gained early experience of a wide range of handicaps in children and adults whilst working in community-based clinics.

She developed her expertise in neurogenic disorders at a joint services rehabilitation unit, where the nature of her caseload necessitated consideration of alternative and augmentative communication methods. Since 1977 she has been involved with the Makaton Vocabulary Development Project, for which she travelled extensively in the UK as part of workshop teams.

In 1979 she joined the staff at the National Hospitals College of Speech Sciences, where she lectured on acquired speech and language disorders. She left to study at California State University, Hayward, USA and was awarded an MA in Communication Processes in December 1985. Her master's thesis considered the differential diagnosis of the hypokinetic dysarthria of Parkinson's disease from other dysarthrias.

On her return to England she joined the staff at the Central School of Speech and Drama as 4th year co-ordinator for the BSc (Hons) Speech and Language Pathology and is responsible for the organization and teaching of the curriculum for acquired neurological disorders.

CHAPTER 1
THE PROBLEM OF DYSARTHRIA

The patient suffering from acquired dysarthria presents a considerable challenge to the student and the qualified speech therapist. He may be distressed and frustrated by his impaired, or total lack of, ability to communicate; he may be depressed by his illness and his weakened physical state; he may lack motivation and tire easily; he may experience a sense of loss of status within his family and society and he may be suffering from a progressive, degenerative, neurological disease.

Such a formidable list of problems is not an exaggeration of the disorders to be faced in a hospital clinic, but rather it is a realistic summary of the problems of many dysarthric patients. Patients whose neurological diagnoses include Parkinson's Disease, Multiple Sclerosis, Pseudobulbar Palsy or Motor Neurone Disease may present just such a list. In addition, one must consider the countless number of brain-damaged patients whose dysarthria is a result of acute trauma, tumour, inflammatory disease or stroke.

Perhaps it is because of the widespread nature of the etiological factors of dysarthria, or the limited positive prognostic expectations in many cases, that medical personnel are often reluctant to refer such patients for speech therapy. This reluctance may be compounded by the speech therapist's own hesitation to engage in a treatment programme with a patient known to have a degenerative condition and therefore a very poor prognosis for return of speech. Whatever the reason may be, the fact remains that many dysarthric patients who could benefit never receive speech therapy. This has a spiral effect in that the fewer the patients who are treated, the less will be the cumulative experience and confidence of therapists; and therefore there will be less evidence of successful therapy. Going full cycle, this could mean a continuance of the reluctance to refer patients in the first instance.

In the field of speech pathology, dysarthria had been for many years a kind of 'Cinderella' in terms of the amount of literature available for study. However, the publication of Darley, Aronson and Brown's book *Motor Speech Disorders* (1975) heralded a new era for those interested in the subject. In this book, the findings of extensive research at the Mayo clinic have helped to give a firm foundation to the theoretical issues concerning the dysarthrias. There has been universal acceptance of their classification system for dysarthria: Flaccid, Spastic, Ataxic, Hypokinetic, Hyperkinetic and Mixed Dysarthria. This system reinforces the clear neuro-anatomical basis on which differential diagnosis may be made.

Darley et al. also clearly identified the wide range of parameters to be considered in relation to dysarthria. These include respiration, phonation, resonance, articulation and prosody. The importance of understanding incompetent valving mechanisms of the air stream was also noted, as was the analysis of the salient neuro-muscular functions involved in motor speech production: strength of muscular contraction; speed of movement; range of excursion of the part being moved; accuracy of movement; steadiness of the contraction and muscular tone.

Thus we now have a firm theoretical core of knowledge of the nature and range of the dysarthrias. However, the current authors' recent experiences have helped to highlight two continuing areas of basic need identified by speech therapists who would have been more willing to tackle the problems of dysarthria if they had additional tools for the job. The first of these needs was for a practical, comprehensive assessment procedure that would adequately identify and describe the range of speech and associated problems of the dysarthric patient. The second was for a compendium of proven, useful exercises and treatment methods to alleviate these problems.

This led to the publication in 1982 of the Robertson Dysarthria Profile. This was the result of six years of research and planning to find a method of assessment that would be an acceptable, practical, clinical tool for therapists. The Profile is based on the theoretical foundations laid down by Darley et al. and consists of sub-tests which are divided into eight areas of assessment. These areas relate to respiration, phonation, facial musculature, diadochokinesis, reflexes, articulation, intelligibility and prosody. The parameters assessed correspond in the main to those identified by Darley as possible areas of disturbance. The Profile also takes cognizance of the features of neuro-muscular functioning of the motor speech system outlined in the Mayo study.

The three main aims of the Profile stated in the manual are that the assessment should provide the practising therapist with '(i) a profile of the patient's abilities and disabilities; (ii) descriptive information to help in classification of the dysarthric problem; and (iii) a sound basis on which to build a therapy and management programme.'

It is hoped that, since its publication, the Dysarthria Profile has achieved the first two of these aims, to some degree at least.

The purpose of this book is to develop the third aim of the Profile. Using the parameters assessed by the Profile it is intended to provide the clinician with some practical suggestions for treatment in these areas. In the main, the suggestions made are based on personal clinical experience and are intended to offer the practising therapist guidelines for therapy which can be developed and expanded according to the ever-changing needs of the individual patient.

It would be folly to suggest that all patients with dysarthria will show great improvement in motor speech production. Many will be suffering from neurological diseases that will bring about either rapid or slow deterioration of their general condition. Many may exhibit an almost pathological lack of motivation or may have been referred for therapy when their condition has already reached a level at which it is almost impossible to treat or alleviate symptoms.

However, it is the authors' firm belief that almost all patients will benefit from a period of therapy, preferably intensive. The results of such therapy may be varied, ranging from considerable improvement or complete recovery of speech processes, to a level of maintenance, albeit of impaired ability to communicate, which may delay to some extent the natural course of the disease. Therapy may also result in the patient's increased ability to analyse and monitor his own speech; to achieve a moderate improvement in his speech; to use techniques designed to help him economize on his efforts to speak; and also, if required, to learn to use augmentative or alternative methods of communication.

CHAPTER 2
BEFORE THERAPY

The Case History

It is widely accepted that adequate case history information is a prerequisite for embarking on a treatment programme for the dysarthric patient.

Knowledge of the medical diagnosis is vital as the severity of the dysarthria is directly related to the site, extent and nature of the lesion, and the prognosis is related to the predicted course of the neurological disease. Information about the site of the lesion will give valuable guidelines to the classification of the dysarthria. In addition, the diagnosis of a specific neurological condition and information relating to the onset and development of symptoms will provide the therapist with vital clues to help in the management of the patient.

If there is a record of neuro-surgical intervention or if a course of medical treatment (eg drugs) has been implemented, then this, too, is vital information for the therapist.

The Assessment

Since 'dysarthria comprises a group of related motor speech disorders' (Darley, 1975; Rosenbek & La Pointe, 1978), a detailed assessment of the range and severity of the speech problem is imperative. It is not only necessary to identify the areas that may be involved, but it is also vital to identify the level at which these problems may occur.

The areas assessed should include: respiratory and phonatory mechanisms; the facility of movement of the speech musculature; articulation; intelligibility and also the suprasegmental, prosodic features of intonation, stress, rhythm and rate.

In relation to the muscles involved in respiration, phonation, articulation and the reflex activities of, for example, chewing, swallowing and coughing, it is important to assess the six properties of neuro-muscular functioning. These properties include muscle strength, speed of movement, range of movement, accuracy of movement, steadiness of contraction and tone. The degree to which these are affected in the different muscle groups will have an important bearing on the severity of the patient's dysarthria and hence the level at which treatment will be focused.

As well as identifying defective functioning, an assessment should also indicate areas of relative strength and less impaired function, as these will be important aspects to consider and utilize in treatment.

The 38 deviant speech dimensions which Darley, Aronson and Brown (1975) identified from the Mayo Study have formed the basis of both formal and informal assessment procedures during the last 10 years. This list of dimensions, however, is basically a check list of possible problem areas and a more sensitive clinical procedure is required to test and hence to identify the strengths and weaknesses of the patient's motor speech abilities.

In 1979 the first edition of the Frenchay Dysarthria Assessment was published (revised edition 1983). This is a useful assessment procedure which helps in particular to diagnose and classify the specific type of dysarthria which may exist.

The author's own assessment, The Dysarthria Profile (1982), which is described in chapter 1, is the assessment which is referred to throughout this text, as one of its main aims is to provide 'a sound basis on which to build a therapy and management programme'.

CHAPTER 3
GENERAL PRINCIPLES AND GOALS OF THERAPY

'Only if a dysarthric patient's nervous system returns to normal will his speech return too. The return to normal— either because of natural or physiologic recovery or because of medical treatment—is a rare circumstance indeed.'

This very realistic observation of Rosenbek and La Pointe (1978) may at first discourage the therapist from even beginning to attempt to treat the patient. However, Rosenbek and La Pointe's optimistic view of dysarthria therapy is revealed in their next statement.

'Therefore the goal of essentially all dysarthria treatment is not normal speech, but compensated intelligibility. With professional guidance and by dint of individual effort, some dysarthric patients can learn to tease or wrench functional speech from their ravaged speech mechanisms.'

It is worth recalling the fundamental principles outlined by Darley, Aronson and Brown (1975), which should form the basis for any therapy programme.
These are:

1. Compensation – the patient learning to maximize the use of his remaining potential

2. Purposeful activity—the patient learning to do 'on purpose' what he has been doing automatically before

3. Monitoring—the patient learning to monitor, check and criticize his own performance

4. An early start—the patient beginning at a very early stage to monitor, practise and compensate before succumbing to inefficient speech habits that are hard to eradicate

5. Motivation—the therapist encouraging the patient to 'embark on and persist in a programme of therapy'.

No matter what the etiology, the type or the severity of dysarthria, these principles should underpin all the clinician's endeavours with the patient.

To these can be added the specific goals for therapy that have been outlined by Rosenbek and La Pointe:

1. helping the patient to become a productive patient

2. modification of posture, muscle tone and strength

3. modification of respiration

4. modification of phonation

5. modification of resonance

6. modification of articulation

7. modification of suprasegmentals and prosody

8. providing alternative modes of communication.

These goals of therapy fit well into the mould of treatment planning suggested by the Dysarthria Profile. The headings used in the following chapters are based on the Profile parameters, but it should be noted that they are closely allied to the above goals. Readers wishing to pursue in depth the Rosenbek goals are referred to: *Clinical Management of Neurogenic Communicative Disorders* edited by Donnell F. Johns (1978).

One further principle which underlies treatment is that 'Dysarthria therapy is drill or the systematic practice of specially selected and ordered exercises' (Rosenbek & La Pointe, 1978). It is important, therefore, to try to impress upon both patients and their relatives that periodic practice sessions should be carried out throughout each day.

Finally, regarding the focus of therapy, Chapter 4 will illustrate the writers' view that one does not treat a specific type of dysarthria (eg. Flaccid, Spastic, Hypokinetic, etc.) or a specific type of neurological disease (eg. Parkinson's Disease, Multiple Sclerosis, Pseudobulbar Palsy). The focus of therapy arises from, firstly, carefully analysing the affected parameters; secondly, grouping these in a logical manner (eg. respiration and phonation; or facial musculature, diadochokinesis and articulation); and thirdly, bearing in mind the underlying pathology and associated physical and psychological factors.

CHAPTER 4

THE PATIENT'S PROFILE

The Dysarthria Profile* is designed to test eight main parameters of motor speech. These parameters are:

1. Respiration

2. Phonation

3. Facial Musculature

4. Diadochokinesis

5. Reflexes

6. Articulation

7. Intelligibility

8. Prosody/Rate.

The method of scoring is both quantitative and qualitative.

The quantitative method is a rating scale with five points—Normal, Good (Adequate), Fair, Poor, Nil. For the most part the tester is required to make a clinical judgement and rate the patient's performance at one of these points. Where a definitive measurement is possible (eg. length of sustaining /a:/—measured with a stop watch in seconds; diadochokinetic rates—measured with a stop watch and digital counter), then this measurement is converted into one of the named points on the rating scale according to the guidance given in the manual.

The qualitative 'score' is really a description of various features of the dysarthria which are not measurable in a quantifiable way. The description, though not 'rateable', provides important information for the clinician who must take all aspects of the patient's profile into consideration when planning therapy.

Information from the quantitative score is collated on a summary form and this provides a simple, quick way to identify the patient's deficits and abilities.

The following two examples will provide the reader with descriptions of the patients' dysarthrias, and also a basis and plan for therapeutic intervention in each case.

Frenchay - Endelby - helps to diagnose & classify specific type of dysarthria.
Robertson - aims to provide sound basis to build on therapy & management.

---

* The Robertson Dysarthria Profile (1982) is available from Winslow Press.

DYSARTHRIA PROFILE — SUMMARY

PATIENTS NAME ...... *JOHN* ......

Hospital No. .... D. of B. *5-2-24* Medical Diagnosis *PARKINSON'S DISEASE*

Physical Condition ...*MOBILE, FIT*........ Date of onset of Dysarthria ...... *1978* ......

Date of Testing ...*1-5-84*... Name of Tester ....

Summary of Type and Severity of Dysarthria ...... *HYPOKINETIC EXTRAPYRAMIDAL* ...... *DYSARTHRIA (MODERATELY SEVERE)* ......

Dates of retest ....

		Normal	Good	Fair	Poor	Nil	TASK	
I.	**RESPIRATION**						1. Sustain /s/ on exhalation	
							2. 'Crescendo' on /s/	
							3. 'Diminuendo' on /s/	
							4. Repeat series of /s/	
							5. Synchronise respiration/phonation	
II.	**PHONATION**						1. Initiate /a:/	
							2. Sustain /a:/	
							3. Say /a:/ loudly	
							4. 'Crescendo' on /a:/	
							5. 'Diminuendo' on /a:/	
							6. Repeat series of /a:/	
							7. Raise pitch on /a:/	
							8. Lower pitch on /a:/	
							9. Glide up scale on /a:/	
							10. Glide down scale on /a:/	
							11. Maintain adequate volume in speech	
							12. Quality of voice	
III.	**FACIAL MUSCULATURE**						1. Symmetry of face at rest	**FACE**
							2. Change expression to smile	
							3. Purse lips	**LIPS**
							4. Stretch lips	
							5. Maintain lip closure at rest	
							6. Achieve lip closure during speech	
							7. Open/close mouth	**JAW**
							8. Move mandible to right	
							9. Move mandible to left	
							10. Protrude tongue	**TONGUE**
							11. Retract tongue	
							12. Move tongue to right	
							13. Move tongue to left	
							14. Pass tongue over teeth	
							15. Move tongue tip into right cheek	
							16. Move tongue tip into left cheek	
							17. Raise tongue tip in mouth	
							18. Raise tongue tip outside mouth	
							19. Elevate soft palate on /a:/	**S.P.**
							20. Elevate soft palate on series of /a:/	

	Normal	Good	Fair	Poor	Nil	TASK
IV. DIADOCHOKINESIS			X			1. Open/Close mouth rapidly
			X			2. Protrude/Retract lips rapidly
			X			3. Protrude/Retract tongue rapidly
				X		4. Elevate /Lower tongue tip rapidly
			X			5. Move tongue side/side rapidly
			X			6. Repeat 'oo–ee' rapidly
	X					7. Repeat 'pa...' rapidly
		X				8. Repeat 'ta...' rapidly
		X				9. Repeat 'ka...' rapidly
		X				10. Repeat 'kala...' rapidly
		X				11. Repeat 'p.t.k...' rapidly
V. REFLEXES	X					1. Chewing
	X					2. Swallow solid food
	X					3. Swallow liquids
	X					4. Prevent drooling at rest
	X					5. Prevent drooling during eating
	X					6. Prevent drooling during speech
	X					7. Cough/clear throat
VI. ARTICULATION	X					1. Repeat initial consonants
	X					2. Accuracy of vowel sounds
	X					3. Repeat consonant clusters
	X					4. Repeat polysyllabic words
	X					5. Repeat phrases
VII. INTELLIGIBILITY		X				1. Intelligibility of reading to therapist
			X			2. Intelligibility of reading to rel/friend
		X				3. Intelligibility of reading to stranger
		X				4. Intelligibility of speech to therapist
			X			5. Intelligibility of speech to rel/friend
		X				6. Intelligibility of speech to stranger
VIII. PROSODY/RATE		X				1. Maintain appropriate rate
		X				2. Increase rate
		X				3. Maintain appropriate rhythm
		X				4. Use appropriate intonation
	X					5. Imitate different stress patterns

7

DYSARTHRIA PROFILE — SUMMARY

PATIENTS NAME .... LAURENCE

Hospital No. .... D. of B. 10-11-61 .... Medical Diagnosis R.T.A. HEAD INJURY

Physical Condition MOBILE, BUT UNSTEADY .... Date of onset of Dysarthria 13-8-83

Date of Testing 1-12-83 .... Name of Tester ....

Summary of Type and Severity of Dysarthria FLACCID DYSARTHRIA (SEVERE)

Dates of retest ....

		Normal	Good	Fair	Poor	Nil	TASK	
I.	RESPIRATION			X			1. Sustain /s/ on exhalation	
				X			2. 'Crescendo' on /s/	
				X			3. 'Diminuendo' on /s/	
			X				4. Repeat series of /s/	
			X				5. Synchronise respiration/phonation	
II.	PHONATION		X				1. Initiate /a:/	
			X				2. Sustain /a:/	
				X			3. Say /a:/ loudly	
				X			4. 'Crescendo' on /a:/	
				X			5. 'Diminuendo' on /a:/	
				X			6. Repeat series of /a:/	
				X			7. Raise pitch on /a:/	
				X			8. Lower pitch on /a:/	
				X			9. Glide up scale on /a:/	
				X			10. Glide down scale on /a:/	
			X				11. Maintain adequate volume in speech	
				X			12. Quality of voice	
III.	FACIAL MUSCULATURE		X				1. Symmetry of face at rest	FACE
			X				2. Change expression to smile	
			X				3. Purse lips	
			X				4. Stretch lips	LIPS
			X				5. Maintain lip closure at rest	
			X				6. Achieve lip closure during speech	
			X				7. Open/close mouth	
			X				8. Move mandible to right	JAW
			X				9. Move mandible to left	
			X				10. Protrude tongue	
			X				11. Retract tongue	
			X				12. Move tongue to right	
			X				13. Move tongue to left	
			X				14. Pass tongue over teeth	TONGUE
			X				15. Move tongue tip into right cheek	
			X				16. Move tongue tip into left cheek	
			X				17. Raise tongue tip in mouth	
			X				18. Raise tongue tip outside mouth	
				X			19. Elevate soft palate on /a:/	S.P.
				X			20. Elevate soft palate on series of /a:/	

		Normal	Good	Fair	Poor	Nil	TASK
IV.	DIADOCHOKINESIS						1. Open/Close mouth rapidly
							2. Protrude/Retract lips rapidly
							3. Protrude/Retract tongue rapidly
							4. Elevate /Lower tongue tip rapidly
							5. Move tongue side/side rapidly
							6. Repeat 'oo—ee' rapidly
							7. Repeat 'pa...' rapidly
							8. Repeat 'ta...' rapidly
							9. Repeat 'ka...' rapidly
							10. Repeat 'kala...' rapidly
							11. Repeat 'p.t.k...' rapidly
V.	REFLEXES						1. Chewing
							2. Swallow solid food
							3. Swallow liquids
							4. Prevent drooling at rest
							5. Prevent drooling during eating
							6. Prevent drooling during speech
							7. Cough/clear throat
VI.	ARTICULA-TION						1. Repeat initial consonants
							2. Accuracy of vowel sounds
							3. Repeat consonant clusters
							4. Repeat polysyllabic words
							5. Repeat phrases
VII.	INTELLIGI-BILITY						1. Intelligibility of reading to therapist
							2. Intelligibility of reading to rel/friend
							3. Intelligibility of reading to stranger
							4. Intelligibility of speech to therapist
							5. Intelligibility of speech to rel/friend
							6. Intelligibility of speech to stranger
VIII.	PROSODY/RATE						1. Maintain appropriate rate
							2. Increase rate
							3. Maintain appropriate rhythm
							4. Use appropriate intonation
							5. Imitate different stress patterns

DYSARTHRIA PROFILE – FORM FOR SCORING

NAME: LAURENCE

D. of B. 10-11-61

MEDICAL DIAGNOSIS: HEAD INJURY

DATE OF TESTING: 1-12-83

Descriptive information (Underline where relevant)

I.

(a) Respiration at rest is: **NORMAL**, SHALLOW
(b) Speed of respiration at rest is: NORMAL, RAPID, **SLOW**
(c) Respiration during speech is: **NORMAL**, SHALLOW
(d) Speed of respiration during speech is: NORMAL, RAPID, **SLOW**
(e) Patient speaks on: **EXHALATION**, INHALATION, **RESIDUAL AIR** (occasionally)
(f) Respiration occurs: **WITHOUT STRIDOR**, WITH STRIDOR

II.

(a) Pitch of voice for speech is: NORMAL, TOO HIGH, **TOO LOW**
(b) Pitch breaks: **DO NOT OCCUR**, DO OCCUR
(c) Intonation for speech is: NORMAL, **MONOTONOUS**, INAPPROPRIATE
(d) Tone of voice is: NORMAL, **HYPERNASAL**, HYPONASAL
(e) Voice quality is: NORMAL, HOARSE, **BREATHY**, **WEAK**, STRIDENT, **INTERMITTENT**

Scoring

	Normal	Good	Fair	Poor	Nil	TASK
I. RESPIRATION			✓			1. Ability to sustain /s/ on exhalation 10 secs.
			✓			2. Ability to 'crescendo' on /s/
			✓			3. Ability to 'diminuendo' on /s/
		✓				4. Ability to repeat series of /s/
			✓			5. Ability to synchronise respiration with phonation
II. PHONATION		✓				1. Ability to initiate /a:/
		✓				2. Ability to sustain /a:/ '3 secs
			✓			3. Ability to say /a:/ very loudly
				✓		4. Ability to 'crescendo' on /a:/
				✓		5. Ability to 'diminuendo' on /a:/
				✓		6. Ability to repeat series of /a:/
				✓		7. Ability to raise pitch on /a:/
				✓		8. Ability to lower pitch on /a:/
				✓		9. Ability to glide up scale on /a:/
				✓		10. Ability to glide down scale on /a:/
				✓		11. Ability to maintain adequate volume in speech
			✓			12. Quality of voice

© ROBERTSON, 1st Edition 1982

1

DESCRIPTIVE INFORMATION

(Head tilts to left)

III.

(a) At rest face: DROOPS ON RIGHT SIDE, **DROOPS ON LEFT SIDE**, MOVES INVOLUNTARILY.

(b) During smile face: DROOPS ON RIGHT SIDE, DROOPS ON LEFT SIDE, MOVES INVOLUNTARILY.

(c) Tone of lips appears: NORMAL, INCREASED, DECREASED. *(in speech)*

(d) At rest tongue appears: **NORMAL**, LARGE, SMALL, FLOPPY, BUNCHED, WASTED, TREMULOUS, FASCICULATING, **FURRED**, WITH FOOD RESIDUE, DEVIATING TO RIGHT, DEVIATING TO LEFT.

(e) Tone of tongue appears: NORMAL, INCREASED, DECREASED.

(f) At rest soft palate is: NORMAL, DEVIATES TO RIGHT, **DEVIATES TO LEFT**. *(slight)*

(g) During phonation soft palate is: NORMAL, DEVIATES TO RIGHT, DEVIATES TO LEFT. *(Rises very slightly.)*

III. FACIAL MUSCULATURE

	TASK	Normal	Good	Fair	Poor	Nil
F A C E	1. Symmetry of facial expression at rest			✓		
	2. Ability to change expression to smile		✓			
L I P S	3. Ability to purse lips			✓		
	4. Ability to stretch lips			✓		
	5. Ability to maintain lip closure at rest		✓			
	6. Ability to achieve lip closure during speech *(weak)*			✓		
J A W	7. Ability to open and close mouth			✓		
	8. Ability to move mandible to right			✓		
	9. Ability to move mandible to left			✓		
T O N G U E	10. Ability to protrude tongue			✓		
	11. Ability to retract tongue		✓			
	12. Ability to move tongue to right		✓			
	13. Ability to move tongue to left		✓			
	14. Ability to pass tongue over teeth			✓		
	15. Ability to move tongue tip into right cheek			✓		
	16. Ability to move tongue tip into left cheek			✓		
	17. Ability to raise tongue tip in mouth		✓			
	18. Ability to raise tongue tip outside mouth		✓			
S. P.	19. Ability to elevate soft palate on /a:/				✓	
	20. Ability to elevate soft palate on series of /a:/				✓	

11

DESCRIPTIVE INFORMATION

IV.

	No. in 5 secs
1. Open/close mouth	9
2. Protrude/retract lips	3
3. Protrude/retract tongue	10
4. Elevate/lower tongue	5–6
5. Lateral tongue	6
6. 'oo ee...'	5
7. 'pa...'	6
8. 'ta...'	7
9. 'ka...'	6
10. 'ka-la...'	4
11. 'p-t-k...'	4

{ very slight movement — note bracketing items 3 & 4 }

TASK

	TASK	Nil	Poor	Fair	Good	Normal
IV. DIADOCHOKINESIS (WITHOUT PHONATION)	1. Ability to open & close mouth rapidly			✓		
	2. Ability to protrude & retract lips rapidly		✓			
	3. Ability to protrude & retract tongue rapidly		✓	✓		
	4. Ability to elevate & lower tongue tip rapidly		✓			
	5. Ability to move tongue rapidly from side to side		✓			
(WITH PHONATION)	6. Ability to repeat 'oo-ee' rapidly			✓		
	7. Ability to repeat 'pa-pa' rapidly		✓			
	8. Ability to repeat 'ta-ta...' rapidly		✓			
	9. Ability to repeat 'ka-ka' rapidly		✓			
	10. Ability to repeat 'ka-la' rapidly		✓			
	11. Ability to repeat 'p-t-k' rapidly			✓		
V. REFLEXES	1. Ability to chew			✓		
	2. Ability to swallow solid food		✓	✓		
	3. Ability to swallow liquids			✓		
	4. Ability to prevent drooling at rest				✓	
	5. Ability to prevent drooling during eating				✓	
	6. Ability to prevent drooling during speech				✓	
	7. Ability to cough/clear throat		✓			

DESCRIPTIVE INFORMATION

VI. 1

Word		Word (3)		(4)	
pie ●	✓	plate ●●	✓	calendar	✓
boy ●	✓	bread ●●	✓	peppermint	✓
tar	✓	tree tɹiː	✓	caterpillar	✓
day	✓	clock ●●	✓	monotonous	✓
car	✓	queen	✓	examination	✓
go ●	✓	grape gɹeɪp	✓	autobiography	✓
four	✓	flower	✓	TOTAL 4/6	
via		frog	✓		
thaw fɔ:	✓	three fɹiː	✓	**(5)**	
the dʒə	✓	spoon	✓	Open the door	✓
sea	✓	smoke	✓	Come in and sit down	✓
zoo	✓	star	✓	Would you like a cup of tea?	✓
shoe	✓	sky	✓	Do you take sugar?	✓
chew	✓	slide	✓	TOTAL 0/4	
jar	✓	splash	✓		
lie	✓	straw stɔː	✓		
roe	✓	scream skiːm	✓		
we	✓	finger	✓		
how	✓	birthday fɛd	✓		
you	✓	lamps læm?	✓		
me	✓	TOTAL 13/20			
no	✓				
TOTAL 16/22					

VIII. (a) Rate of speech is: NORMAL, **TOO SLOW,** TOO FAST, FESTINATES, SLOWS DOWN.

(b) Rhythm of speech is: NORMAL, SYLLABIC, STACCATO, WITH PROLONGATIONS, **WITH INSUFFICIENT STRESSING.**

● weak plosives (also weak fricatives)
●● slow laboured articulation

		TASK	Normal	Good	Fair	Poor	Nil
VI. ARTICULATION	1.	Ability to repeat initial consonants			✓		
	2.	Accuracy of vowel sounds (nasalized)				✓	
	3.	Ability to repeat consonant clusters			✓		
	4.	Ability to repeat polysyllabic words				✓	
	5.	Ability to repeat phrases					✓
VII. INTELLIGIBILITY	1.	Intelligibility of reading to therapist				✓	
	2.	Intelligibility of reading to relative/friend				✓	
	3.	Intelligibility of reading to stranger				✓	
	4.	Intelligibility of speech to therapist				✓	
	5.	Intelligibility of speech to relative/friend				✓	
	6.	Intelligibility of speech to stranger				✓	
VIII. PROSODY/RATE	1.	Ability to maintain appropriate rate				✓	
	2.	Ability to increase rate				✓	
	3.	Ability to maintain appropriate rhythm				✓	
	4.	Ability to use appropriate intonation				✓	
	5.	Ability to imitate different stress patterns				✓	

13

Profile I: John

Interpreting John's Profile

1. First refer to Section VII (Intelligibility) for an overall view of the severity of John's problem. His wife (the relative in this case) is able to understand him adequately (GOOD) in both reading and conversation. However the therapist and strangers find him more difficult to understand (FAIR) in both these situations.

2. Is John's impaired intelligibility due to poor articulation? Refer to Section VI (Articulation). There is apparently no real deficit whatsoever in this area, other than a slight reduction of accuracy in repetition of phrases. (The accuracy of John's articulation is linked with the overall adequacy of movement of the facial musculature (Section III); his intact reflexes (Section V); and the fairly adequate diadochokinetic rates of movement for the repetition of different phonemes (Section IV).) The rather strange pattern of diado-chokinetic rates, where the movements without phonation are not as good as the movements with phonation, is not unusual in Parkinson's Disease. In this type of case great variation is found, particularly where there is either bradykinesia or festinance.

3. What, therefore, is the cause of John's impaired intelligibility? A glance at the Phonation, Respiration and Prosody Sections (II, I and VIII) indicates the probable source of the problem. All aspects of voicing score at a maximum level of FAIR while changing pitch and varying intonation score as POOR (cf. monotony of voice, typical of Hypokinetic Dysarthria). These problems of phonation are closely linked with and probably caused by the respiratory problems of poor capacity, control and synchronization with phonation. The respiratory and phonatory problems are probably contributory factors in the lack of appropriate use of rhythm and intonation, identified in the Prosody Section (VIII).

Focus of Therapy

Therapy for John will be focused in three main areas: Respiration, Phonation and Prosody. Because of their relationship to each other they should be treated in this order. In other words, since Prosody is totally dependent on adequate voicing and breath control, it should be treated last. Since respiratory control is the foundation of good phonation, then breathing exercises to establish adequate method, capacity and control of respiration should precede exercises which involve production, control and variation of voice.

Profile 2: Laurence

Interpreting Laurence's Profile

1. Again, first refer to Section VII (Intelligibility) for an overall view of the severity of Laurence's problem. This indicates that Laurence has a very severe problem, as *everyone* who comes into contact with him has great difficulty understanding him (POOR).

2. Is Laurence's poor intelligibility due to impaired articulation? Examination of Section VI (Articulation) indicates a real problem in this area. Production of consonants is fairly poor and vowel production shows an even greater deficit. His difficulties are most marked when attempting polysyllabic words and phrases.

3. Is Laurence's poor articulation due to impaired movement of the facial musculature? Section III (Facial Musculature), Section IV (Diadochokinesis) and Section V (Reflexes) all indicate deficits. Section III provides the information that, with the exception of the soft palate, all the other articulatory organs have the potential for movement. However, Sections V and VI would suggest sluggishness, slowness and overall lack of competence in speed and co-ordination of movement both at a reflex level and at the level of voluntary control.

4. It is of particular relevance to consider the poor performance of the soft palate (Section III, Subtests 19, 20 and Descriptive Information III, points f, g). The velum appears to move minimally and results in obvious inadequacy of naso-pharyngeal valving which is probably the cause of the poor voice quality (Section III, Subtest 12); the hypernasality (Descriptive Information, II, point d) and the distorted vowels (Section VI, Subtest 2).

5. An examination of Section II (Phonation) indicates a severe problem of voice production, mainly in relation to variation of volume, pitch and intonation, rather than in initiating or sustaining phonation. Here, the reduced ability to control respiration (Section I) and to synchronize respiration and phonation are probably contributory factors.

6. The combined effects of poor respiration, phonation, and articulation almost certainly result in totally inadequate prosody and rate (Section VIII) and this in turn compounds the problem of lack of intelligibility.

Focus of Therapy

Therapy for Laurence must take into account *all* the parameters involved in speech production. Control of respiration and its co-ordination with phonation will certainly require attention.

However, probably the most essential area to work on initially is that of the oro-facial musculature. The strength, range and speed of tongue and lip movements in particular must be highlighted. In addition, exercises or a prosthetic device should be given to try to alleviate the problem of poor soft palate movement.

When control of respiration and phonation have improved and when adequate speed and co-ordination of the oro-facial musculature have been achieved, then therapy can proceed to systematic articulation practice, building up from sounds in isolation, clusters, single syllables, to polysyllabic words, then phrases and sentences.

During the latter stages of articulation work, the prosodic variations of stress, intonation, rhythm and rate can be introduced and practised.

Chapter 5
RELAXATION

Boone (1983) considers relaxation to mean 'a realistic responsiveness to the environment with a minimum of needless energy expended'. Many dysarthric patients show signs of excessive body tension and, in Boone's terms, this means that they are expending energy which could be utilized positively.

The damaging effects of tension upon the laryngeal and pharyngeal musculature are evident in vocal strain and this is also apparent in many dysarthric patients. Merely drawing attention to the existence of tension does not often result in the patient controlling this, particularly in relation to the laryngeal structures and the tongue. Jacobson (1957) has found that the involuntary muscles of the body become relaxed as the voluntary groups are freed from residual tension. Therefore it would seem that, in order to reduce tension in the speech mechanism, it is justifiable and logical to work from a basis of general relaxation of the whole body.

Approaches

There are two approaches to relaxation therapy:

1. A direct, physical approach, using a series of structured exercises to encourage a progressive state of relaxation.

2. Relaxation through suggestion. This may be physical suggestion (eg. 'Your arm is limp and heavy and is hanging loosely') or through the use of mental imagery. Moncur and Brackett (1974) point out that in behaviour therapy, the presentation of pleasurable scenes to a client is used extensively to induce a sense of well-being and relaxation. It has been found that relaxation is usually achieved in less time with scene presentation than with most other methods.

Whichever method of relaxation is chosen, the therapist is advised to plan in advance of the session to ensure:

(i) that there are no interruptions at the door (a 'Do Not Disturb' sign on the door may suffice)

(ii) that there are no telephone calls (either take the telephone off the hook or redirect calls via secretary/operator)

(iii) that the furniture in the room is arranged appropriately, so that there is a minimum amount of upheaval when the patient enters the room.

Throughout the whole session the therapist must be aware of her own approach to the patient and should create an atmosphere of calm with complete lack of tension. The pitch, tone and speed of the therapist's voice and speech is vital. She should speak in a quiet, relaxed, low pitched voice and at a considerably slower than normal speed. She should repeat instructions when necessary, always maintaining the quiet, relaxed, unruffled atmosphere.

1. Direct Approach

Since the 1930s, the principles of Jacobson's method of progressive relaxation have been used in speech and voice training. However, the procedures are modified to suit the needs of the individual patient. Moncur believes that because speech clinicians commonly use short sessions, the contrasts between tension and relaxation are stressed; whereas they should work for prolonged periods in order to obtain deep relaxation in a specific muscle group. Progressive relaxation enables the patient to become aware of the states of tension and relaxation in the muscle groups and to experience and identify the sensation of relaxation, so that he is able to assess his own responses.

There is often discussion about whether relaxation exercises should take place in a supine position or on a chair. To some extent the decision can be based purely on personal preference, the patient's mobility and the suitability of the clinic surroundings.

Begin by explaining to the patient why relaxation is important and how you intend to proceed. Suggest that he finds a comfortable position. Ask him to clear his mind of other thoughts and to concentrate only on the activities you describe for him to carry out.

(a) Relaxation of feet, legs and buttocks

1. Ask the patient to curl up his toes as tightly as possible . . . hold for 3 seconds . . . and then to release them. Repeat this several times, pointing out that the release enables his legs to relax and loosen too.

2. Follow on, by asking the patient to rotate his ankles, one at a time . . . and then relax.

3. If the patient is in a sitting position, ask him to place his feet flat on the floor and to push 'through' the floor as hard as possible . . . hold for 3 seconds . . . and then relax. Repeat and point out to the patient the tension and relaxing he should be feeling in the calf muscles of his legs.

4. Ask the patient to straighten his legs and to make them 'stiff' at the knees . . . hold for 3 seconds . . . and then relax. Repeat and encourage the patient to feel the tension and relaxing in the knees.

5. Ask the patient to push his thighs and buttocks into the seat of the chair or the couch, to tighten . . . hold for 3 seconds . . . and then relax. Repeat and encourage patient to feel the tension and relaxing of these muscles.

6. Remind the patient that he should now feel that 'all the power' has gone from his feet, legs, knees, thighs and buttocks and that they should all be very relaxed.

7. Before moving on, gently lead into the next stage by saying: 'We are now going to concentrate on your stomach, chest and back, but I want you to maintain the loose feeling in your feet, legs and buttocks.'

(b) Relaxation of stomach, chest and back

1. Ask the patient to pull in and tighten his stomach muscles . . . hold for 3 seconds . . . and then release. Repeat this several times, asking him to become aware of the tension in his back, chest and diaphragm, whilst holding the stomach tight. Urge him to be aware of the contrasting relaxed feeling when he lets go.

2. Encourage the patient to breathe gently and deeply as he relaxes the muscles.

3. Before moving on, again tell the patient that you are now going to concentrate on the arms and hands, but you want him to continue to feel the relaxation in his feet, legs, buttocks, stomach, chest and back.

(c) Relaxation of hands and arms

1. Ask the patient to clench his fists tightly, hold the position and then let go. Repeat this several times.

2. Ask the patient then to raise both arms out in front of him to shoulder height (or waist level if more appropriate) . . . hold for 3 seconds . . . and then let them drop by his side or on to his lap. Repeat this.

3. Then combine these two. Ask the patient to raise his arms and at the same time, clench his fists tightly. Hold this tense position for 3 seconds and then drop the arms and release the fists. Repeat this several times.

4. Repeatedly stress the contrast between the feeling of tension and the feeling of relaxation.

5. If the hands still appear tense, ask the patient to shake each hand gently from the wrist until they feel loose.

6. Before proceeding to the shoulders, head and neck, check that the patient is really aware of the tension and release in those parts of the body you have been working on. Observe for yourself whether the patient is more relaxed now or whether he has returned to his habitual tension pattern. If this is the case, remind him of the exercises you have worked through . . . ask him to focus on each part of the body in turn...and ask him to breathe gently and deeply.

7. You may find it useful, in monitoring the degree of relaxation achieved, to lift the patient's wrist, shake it gently and then let go. You may also raise the patient's arm by lifting at the elbow and then gently let go. The arm will fall down loosely if it is relaxed. (It is important to comment to the patient on what you are doing in the same calm, relaxed tone, so that the patient does not immediately tense when he feels a touch on his wrist or elbow etc.)

8. When he appears to be tension free, talk of moving on to the shoulders, neck and head.

(d) Relaxation of shoulders, neck and head

1. Ask the patient to tense his shoulders tightly in a shrug . . . hold for 3 seconds . . . and then release. Repeat this several times.

2. Ask the patient to drop his head slowly forwards and then gently backwards, then slowly roll his head from one side to the other. Then ask the patient to rotate his head slowly forwards on to his chest, across to the right shoulder, back across to the left shoulder and forward on to the chest again. Do this exercise clockwise first (to right shoulder) and then anti-clockwise (to left shoulder)

to avoid dizziness. This exercise should be done very slowly and gently, as the patient may have some pain and/or limited movement because of eg. arthritis. Closing the eyes may help to avoid a feeling of dizziness.

3. To ensure these head movements are smooth and gentle, it may help to support the patient's head and assist the appropriate movements. Stand behind the patient and place one hand under his chin and the other at the back of his head. By gently pushing alternately on the back of his head and under his chin it is possible to assist the forwards and backwards movements.

4. By changing one's hand positions to support the sides of the patient's head over his ears or by placing one hand under his chin, it is possible to assist the side to side movements.

5. By placing one hand over each of the patient's ears, it is possible to assist the rotating movements.

6. Ask the patient to raise his eyebrows and wrinkle his forehead tightly and then relax. Repeat and feel the difference between tension and relaxation.

7. Ask the patient to clench his jaw, push his lips together and press his tongue hard against the roof of his mouth . . . hold for 3 seconds . . . relax and allow the jaw to drop, the lips to part and the tongue to move slowly away from the hard palate. Repeat.

8. Ask the patient to move his lower jaw very slowly and gently from side to side and then to rotate it gently. This will often result in a yawn.

9. Ask the patient to screw up his face as tightly as possible . . . hold for 3 seconds . . . then relax. Repeat several times.

The purpose of outlining these exercises is to show that it is possible to move systematically through the body and encourage the patient to experience the sensation of relaxation by contrasting the feelings of tension and release in different parts of the body.

This exercise routine need not be too rigidly adhered to. It is possible to vary the exercises by introducing more graded steps. It may also be necessary to spend more time on one area that may be a focus of tension in a particular patient. The important factor is speed: these exercises must be carried out slowly and calmly with the therapist maintaining a relaxed, appropriate voice level.

If the patient has grasped some of the essentials of relaxation during the clinic session, it is very beneficial if he can continue practising at home. A tape recording (eg. of the actual session or the therapist 'talking through' the routine) may be made for the patient to take home and play back each day to guide him through. Alternatively, the patient could play a recording of soft, relaxing music as a background for his home practice.

As the patient progresses, he may be encouraged to use appropriate odd moments of the day to try out some selective relaxation exercises. For example, sitting in the bus or ambulance; when sitting at his desk at work during a coffee break, or when watching television in the evening; or on first lying down in bed at night.

2. Suggestion

It is possible to 'set a scene' which will help to relax the patient immediately or after a series of tensing/relaxing exercises. When using this method, it is important that the patient is aware at all times of what the therapist is trying to help him achieve.

As before, external stimuli should be controlled, so that the patient is not distracted by the telephone ringing or people entering or leaving the room. The patient should be seated comfortably with his eyes closed and should be encouraged to imagine the scene described.

The scenes presented should be tranquil and passive rather than lively or active. In describing a scene as many sensory details as possible should be included—visual, auditory, kinaesthetic, tactile and olfactory.

In describing a warm summer's day in the country, conjure up a picture of the warmth of the sun, the slight swish of the gentle breeze, the sound of the birds and the water in the stream, the smell of the woodland flowers and hedgerows, the feel of the springy grass, the colours of the trees and flowers and the shimmering sunlight on the water etc.

Approximately fifteen to twenty minutes will be necessary for the first session. The amount of time required may be reduced in future sessions as the patient learns to respond more easily to the suggestion.

Presentation of short, pleasant scenes to inhibit negative emotion should be based on information provided by the patient. Ask the patient what are the most pleasant scenes he can imagine, after which it may only be necessary to suggest some sensory features to make the scene more vivid. The patient's own imagination should supply the rest.

Another method of evoking pleasant memories for the patient is to show him pictures of favourite places, people or events. Ask him then to close his eyes and imagine the scene; the therapist again needs add only minimal imagery to elaborate the picture.

Having achieved a state of relaxation of body and mind, the patient can then be moved gently on to active participation (eg. breathing and voicing exercises) but *care must be taken to ensure that the feeling of relaxation remains throughout the rest of the session.*

CHAPTER 6
RESPIRATION

Posture

'Speaking is done most efficiently during standing, sitting, or lying on one's back, so the spine is straight and the head is in a straight line with the body's midline.' (Rosenbek & La Pointe, 1978). Although normal speakers can talk in almost any position, the dysarthric speaker will normally need to find the optimum posture to provide the best background for adequate respiration, phonation and articulation. 'Therefore, an early clinical task is to analyse the dysarthric speaker's posture and decide whether or not to modify it.' (Rosenbek & La Pointe).

The writers quoted above advocate that in some cases specific aids to posture may be adapted for individual patients. A range of supports, slings and braces are described to help compensate for weakness of the neck or limb muscles, for example.

In general, patients should be trained to adopt good posture of the head, neck and trunk. Care should be taken that the patient's body is well supported, normally in an armchair, so that he is able to maintain an upright, symmetrical position. A physiotherapist's observations may be helpful at this stage.

Respiration

The volume and control of the expiratory air column is generally considered to be the basis of correct phonation and it is recognized that no improvement of faulty voice production can be achieved without careful attention to breath control. Good breath support allows for control of loudness of the voice without undue effort. Cooper (1977) further suggests that concentration on breath control takes the muscular tension away from the laryngeal and pharyngeal areas and re-directs it to the abdominal muscles and the diaphragm, which are more able to bear the pressure and tension without interfering with vocalization. The report of Gordon, Morton and Simpson (1978) relating to airflow measurement in diagnosis, assessment and treatment of mechanical dysphonia further confirms the fact that air support in phonation is dependent upon volume and regulation of exhaled air.

As we have seen in a patient's profile in Chapter 4 (John), poor respiration may prove to be the fundamental problem from which all the other motor speech problems arise. Adequate supply and control of exhaled breath is vital to the production of a good quality voice and correct realizations of phonemes. It is also an important prerequisite of good intonation, stressing, rhythm and phrasing. The difference between intelligible and unintelligible speech may indeed arise from the adequacy of the breath source.

The Aims of Respiration Therapy are:

1. To establish the correct breathing pattern (intercostal diaphragmatic)

2. To increase the vital capacity of the lungs

3. To facilitate the control of inhalation and exhalation

4. To improve the strength and the co-ordination of the respiratory muscles

All these exercises should normally be carried out following on from relaxation exercises and should be approached in a calm, methodical manner so that an easy, relaxed atmosphere is maintained. It is important not to rush any of the stages. The therapist should demonstrate each exercise several times and should help the patient to monitor his performance throughout.

Although it may seem tedious to spend a number of sessions on breathing exercises, the establishing of an easy, rhythmical, controlled pattern of respiration will form the basis upon which many of the other therapeutic tasks can be built. Inadequate emphasis and practice at this level may reduce the effectiveness of subsequent therapy; while constant reinforcement of good breath control will lead to a solid foundation for phonation, articulation and prosodic exercises.

The amount of time within each session that should be spent on breathing exercises will vary, not only according to the individual needs of the patient but also the patient's tendency to tire and/or lose concentration. For some patients a five-minute session on these exercises will be sufficient, whereas other patients may be able to attempt a whole range of the exercises for up to 15 or 20 minutes at a time.

Exercises

Respiration Therapy

I Demonstrate to the patient where he should place his hands so as to feel the movement of the diaphragm during respiration (ie. one hand over the diaphragm and the other placed against the lower ribs at the side).

If the patient is unable to use his own hands (eg. because of paralysis), the therapist may stand behind him and place one of her hands over the patient's diaphragm and the other over the lower ribs at one side, or she may hold both hands over the lower rib cage at each side.

It is useful for both the patient and the therapist to stand in front of a mirror during these exercises.

2 Instruct the patient to breathe in gently and easily through the nose and breathe out slowly through the mouth. Note the outwards movement of the diaphragm and the upwards and outwards movement of the ribs. Correct any shoulder movement. Repeat several times, taking care to allow the patient to pause between each deep breath so as to avoid the danger of hyperventilation.

3 Instruct the patient to breathe in whilst the therapist counts to three; to hold his breath to the therapist's count of three; and finally to breathe out slowly through the mouth to the therapist's count of three.

Repeat several times, maintaining breathing in to a count of three and holding to a count of three, but extending the breathing out time to a count of four, then five, then six, and so on up to ten. Ensure that the patient has established a rhythmic pattern, with visible movement of diaphragm and lower ribs, but without shoulder movement.

Continue the exercise without the therapist counting but with the patient monitoring himself by counting silently.

4 Instruct the patient to breathe in to a silent count of three and then exhale breath on a voiceless fricative sound. Begin with /h/ then use the voiceless fricatives /s, /ʃ, /f, θ / in turn.

Monitor the patient's ability to sustain voiceless fricatives by using a stop watch. Aim to achieve eventually, approximately 20 seconds on /s/, but rather less on the other sounds over the course of several sessions.

Where a patient finds difficulty in sustaining /s/ for this period of time after several weeks of practice, accept his maximum level and adjust future therapy accordingly.

5 Continue the previous exercise, but encourage the patient to 'diminuendo' and 'crescendo' on exhaled sound (ie. decrease and increase the intensity of the fricatives).

eg. (i)   SSSSSSSsss

   (ii)   sssSSSSSSSS

   (iii)   sssSSSSSSsss

   (iv)   sssSSSSSsssSSSSSSsss

Repeat this exercise with as many variations as possible on one breath. Encourage the patient to feel the considerable movement and pressure in the area of the diaphragm, which indicates the ability to exert control over the outgoing air stream.

Repeat the exercise over the course of several sessions, gradually introducing the use of the other voiceless fricatives /ʃ, f, θ/.

6 Instruct the patient to practise exhalation of voiceless fricatives in a rhythmic pattern.

Begin by using the /s/ [— indicates a long sound and – indicates a short sound].

eg. /s/ (i)   —— – – —— – – ——
     (ii)   – – —— – – —— – – ——
     (iii)   – —— – —— – —— – ——
     (iv)   —— – – – —— – – – —— – – –

Repeat this exercise introducing as many variations of rhythm as possible. See that the patient repeats each series on a single breath. Repeat the exercise over the course of several sessions, gradually introducing the use of the other voiceless fricatives /ʃ/, f, θ/.

7 Instruct the patient to practise sustaining exhalation on a voiceless, 'whispered' vowel sound. Sustain each sound as long as possible.

Begin with /a:/ then introduce other vowels in turn /u:, ɔ:, i:, ɜ:/, etc.

Repeat this exercise and encourage the patient to link whispered vowel sounds together, followed by combinations of voiceless fricatives and voiceless vowel sounds.

eg. (i)   /a:i:/; / ɔ:u:/; / ɔ:i:/; /u: ɜ :/

   (ii)   /a:i:u:/; / ɔ:a:u:/; /i:u:ɜ:/

   (iii)   /fa: fi: fu: f ɔ:/

   (iv)   /sa: fa: θa: ʃa:/

8 Instruct the patient to hold his lips together in a fairly relaxed position, then blow the lips apart with strong puffs of air, avoiding excessive tension or pressure. Sounds made should resemble voiceless c.v. combinations.

           /pʌpʌpʌpʌ/;   /pæpæpæpæ/;   /pəpəpəpə

Note the intra-oral air pressure just prior to release of air. Look in a mirror and note the bulging of the cheeks and the pouting of the lips.

9 Instruct the patient to practise exhalation on a slow, whispered count of three, gradually increasing the count to ten if possible, in one breath.

eg. (i)   1 – 2 – 3

   (ii)   1 – 2 – 3 – 4

   (iii)   1 – 2 – 3 – 4 – 5

   (iv)   1 – 2 – 3 – 4 – 5 – 6 … 10

10 Repeat the previous exercise but vary the intensity of the whispering (as in exercise 5).

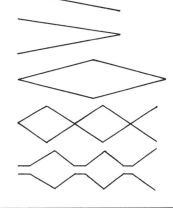

eg. (i)   ₁₂3**45**

   (ii)   **12** 3₄₅

   (iii)   ₁2**34**₅

   (iv)   ₁**2**₃**4**₅**6**

   (v)   ₁₂3₄₅6₇₈**9**

CHAPTER 7
PHONATION

'The main laryngeal movement abnormalities in the dysarthrias are hyperadduction, as in spastic dysarthria; hypoadduction as in flaccid dysarthria and poorly co-ordinated laryngeal movements, as in ataxic dysarthria'. (Rosenbek and La Pointe, 1978).

The focus of therapy for phonation will therefore depend on the type of problem that has been identified during assessment. For example, the patient who has a cerebellar lesion and presents with an ataxic dysarthria is likely to have particular difficulties in initiating phonation and in controlling the loudness and pitch of his voice. Of the exercises which follow, therefore, numbers 1, 2, 8, 14, 15 and 18 may be found to be beneficial. On the other hand a patient with Parkinson's Disease, and hence a probable hypokinetic type of dysarthria, will normally have problems of reduced loudness and monotony of pitch. He may also experience difficulty in initiating phonation. Exercises 1, 2, 4, 5, 7, 8, 9 to 19 will probably be of most benefit to him. The exercises that follow should be selected carefully and used as appropriate to the individual patient's problems.

Aims of Phonation Therapy are:

1. To establish good co-ordination of respiration and phonation

2. To achieve an appropriate vocal 'attack' (neither too hard nor too weak)

3. To control loudness

4. To achieve optimum pitch

5. To facilitate variation of pitch and inflection

6. To achieve appropriate resonance and projection

Exercises for phonation should be linked with work on respiration control in such a way that there is a smooth transition from respiration to phonation. If this does not happen there is a tendency for the patient to think: 'Now we've finished with breathing and we're working on voice'. The therapist must continually remind the patient of the logical progression of these exercises and the need to build upon and extend the breathing exercises.

Aids to Therapy

In exercises aimed at facilitating control and variation of phonation, the use of audio tape recording and/or video taping is recommended. In addition, the laryngograph, spectrographic display, visispeech or visipitch, where available, will be useful adjuncts to therapy. The patient's own perception of his voice may be distorted and he may not be aware of the problems. The introduction of audio recording and visual display facilities should increase his own awareness; and careful and sensitive use of these facilities by the therapist will help him to monitor and improve his performance.

Exercises

Initiation of voice

1   To facilitate initiation of voice and reduce hard attack, instruct the patient to breathe out and sustain the voiceless /h/ with the mouth wide open and then start phonating /aː/. Repeat this exercise several times, gradually reducing the length of the /h/ and increasing the length of the vocalized /aː/.

     eg.   (i) /hhhh .... aː ..../
               (ii) /hhh .... aː ..../
               (iii) /hh .... aː ..../
               (iv) /haː ..../
               (v) /aː................/

Vary this exercise by changing the vowel sound:

     eg.   (i) /h .... uː/
               (ii) /h .... ɔː/
               (iii) /h .... iː/

2   When the patient has mastered the previous exercise, encourage the same approach with different voiceless fricative sounds preceding the vocalized vowels.

     eg.   (i) /s .... aː ; s .... iː ; s .... uː/
               (ii) /ʃ .... aː ; ʃ .... iː ; ʃ .... uː/
               (iii) /f .... aː ; f .... iː ; f .... uː/

3   Where harsh attack is a symptom of extreme laryngeal tension Moncur and Brackett (1974) recommend massage and relaxation techniques. Massage may take the form of manual or vibratory massage in the area of geniohyoid, mylohyoid and digastric muscles. Following massage, there should be a reduction of laryngeal tension making it possible to practise the production of vowels, then syllables.

4 The patient who has a flaccid dysarthria and some degree of laryngeal adductor paralysis should be considered a candidate for some degree of pushing exercises. These exercises are described in detail by Froeschel et al, and reported by Rosenbek and La Pointe (1978). Greene (1980) also discusses methods of achieving voice in such cases.

Instruct the patient to either:

(i) Raise his clenched fists to the level of his chest and then push down suddenly and expel air loudly, or

(ii) Raise his hands to chest level and push palms against the wall in a sudden action as above, or

(iii) Press the palms of the hand firmly and suddenly down on a table or on the arms of the chair, or

(iv) Raise the arms to shoulder level, bent at elbow, lock the fingers of each hand together and try to pull the hands apart in a sudden strong movement.

In all cases the patient should expel air loudly in a 'grunt' and then attempt to continue the vocalization to produce a vowel sound.

eg. /a: ; u: ; i: ; ɔ:/

5 One further method to facilitate initiation of phonation is to ask the patient to take a deep breath and attempt to cough on the outgoing breath and then to 'shape' this vocalization into a vowel sound as indicated above. Once phonation has been established the patient should be encouraged to use a loud sigh in preference to coughing to facilitate voicing, so that there is no habitual use of hard glottal attack.

6 Voiced plosives may also be used to aid initiation of voice.

eg. /ba: ; bu: ; dɔ: ; di:/

Sustaining voice

Once the patient is able to initiate voice appropriately and consistently, the therapist should proceed to encourage sustained voicing. Instruct the patient to sustain a vowel sound on an unbroken breath for an increasing length of time:

eg. /a:/ ; /u:/ ; /i:/ ; / ɜ:/

Monitor the patient's performance by using a stop watch and aim for sustained vocalization of 15 to 20 seconds.

Repeat these exercises in a variety of ways:

eg. Glide from one vowel sound to another within one breath:

(i) /a:u:/ ; /i:ɔ:/ ; /u:ɜ:/ ; /i:u:/

(ii) /a:u:i:/ ; /i:ɜ:ɔ:/ ; /u:i:ɔ:/

When the patient is able to initiate and also sustain phonation it is then possible to move on to a variety of exercises that will facilitate control of a number of aspects of the voice, including projection volume pitch and intonation.

Projection and volume control

1   Instruct the patient on how to produce a sustained humming
    sound /mm .../ . (The lips should make very light contact,
    while the teeth remain apart and the oral cavity is as wide as
    possible behind closed lips. Think the voice forward on to the
    lips, so that the vibration is felt and the sound is not
    constricted back in the pharynx.)

2   When humming is mastered ask the patient to add a
    vocalized vowel sound to the humming. Begin by using the
    most open vowels and then proceed to the closed vowels.

    eg.   (i) /m .... a: ..../ ; /m .... ɜ : .... /; /m .... ɔ: ..../;
                /m .... i: ..../ ; /m .... u: ..../

            (ii) /m .... a: .... m .... ɔ : .... m .... i:/
                 /m .... ɜ : .... m .... u: .... m .... i:/

    Gradually shorten the length of the /m/ and increase the
    length of the vowel sounds.

    eg.   (i) /ma: .... ma: .... ma: ..../
                /mi : .... mi : .... mi : ..../

            (ii) /ma: .... mɔ: .... mɜ: ..../
                 /mi : .... mu: .... mɔ: ..../

3   If a patient finds it difficult to maintain lip contact for the
    bilabial /m/, encourage him to follow the above exercises
    using the alveolar nasal /n/. The additional use of /n/ may
    also add variety for all patients and provide extra practice to
    encourage voice projection.

4 Extend the practice of sustaining and projecting the voice by asking the patient to 'intone' on words and alliterative phrases using combinations of nasal and oral sounds. The object is to achieve good projection and volume of voice and variation of mouth posture to facilitate the contrasts and resonance of the vowel sounds.

eg.   (i) Man, moon, mine, mince,
             money, many, morning, manage,
             minimum, management, marmalade.

        (ii) My mum makes mince on Mondays.
            Many men make much money.
            Martin has marmalade in the morning.
            Mandy likes mince and minestrone soup.
            Management lend minimum money.

5 Using the same style of intoned phonation, ask the patient to recite:

      (i) days of the week
     (ii) months of the year
   (iii) numbers 1 to 20

Make sure that the patient understands the concept of the almost continuous voicing required, with no breaks between words. Make it clear exactly when he should pause, breathe and begin again – eg. after every three words when reciting the days or the months and after every five numbers when counting.

6 To encourage the use of maximum volume in these exercises above, it is suggested that the therapist moves gradually further and further away from the patient until they are as far apart as the size of the room will allow. Encourage the patient to 'fill the room with sound'. (At this point it is important to make sure there is no increase in tension – eg. in posture. If there is, the therapist should remind the patient to remain as relaxed as possible and to breathe as deeply and easily as he can.)

7 To facilitate control of the volume of phonation, ask the patient to repeat the serials indicated in exercise 5 with some variations:

eg.   (i) Count and gradually increase the volume:

1, 2, 3, 4, 5, 6, 7, 8, 9, 10   <

(ii) Count and gradually decrease the volume:

1, 2, 3, 4, 5, 6, 7, 8, 9, 10   >

(iii) Count and increase the volume on every 2nd, 3rd, 4th, 5th number:

(a) 1, 2, 3, 4, 5, 6 . . .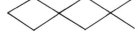

(b) 1, 2, 3, 4, 5, 6, 7, 8, 9 . . .

(c) 1, 2, 3, 4, 5, 6, 7, 8, 9, 10, 11, 12 . . .

(iv) A variation on the above exercise is for the patient and therapist to engage in a kind of dialogue (from opposite ends of the room perhaps), taking it in turn to complete the series with the loud number.

eg.   (a) T = 1, 2, 3, 4   (soft)

P = 5   (loud)

T = 6, 7, 8, 9   (soft)

P = 10   (loud)

(b) T = 1   (soft)

P = 2   (loud)

T = 3   (soft)

P = 4   (loud)

8 Use of a simple sustained phonated vowel may facilitate the control of volume. Ask the patient to sustain the vowel.

(/a:/; /ɔ:/; /i:/; /u:/; etc.)

and to get louder or softer as instructed.

eg.   (i) /a: ....../

(soft → loud)

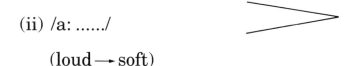

(ii) /a: ....../

(loud → soft)

(iii) /a: ....../

(soft → loud → soft)

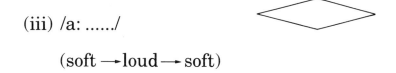

(iv) /a: ....../

(soft → loud → soft → loud → soft → loud)

9 A further exercise to facilitate control of initiation, sustaining, and volume is to ask the patient to produce a series of vowel sounds in different rhythmic patterns.

eg.   Using the sounds /a:/ or /i:/ or /u:/ etc, repeat the following rhythms in a single breath [── represents a long sound and – represents a short sound].

/a:/

(i) – – – – – – – – – –
(ii) ── ── ── ──
(iii) – ── – ── – ── – – ──
(iv) ── – – ── – – – – ──
(v) – – – ── ── ── – – ── ── ──

Pitch and inflection control

Since many dysarthric patients will present with either monotonous voices, or pitch levels that are abnormally high or abnormally low, it is important to try a) to extend the pitch range and facilitate movement from one pitch level to another; *and* b) to help the patient find his optimum pitch and to stabilize his phonation at this level.

Many of the conventional, well established voice exercises will help to realize these two objectives.

To extend the pitch range, encourage the patient to sing up and down the scale. Use any vowel or consonant/vowel combination that the patient finds easy, eg, /la: la: la:/; /ma: ma: ma:/; /a: a: a:/; /bi: bi: bi:/; /dɔ: dɔ: dɔ:/ etc.

If the patient is unable to sing a whole octave, concentrate on trying to achieve three different pitches: low/middle/high. Then try to extend his range gradually over the course of several sessions. The use of a tuning fork and/or xylophone may help the therapist and patient to monitor how many changes of pitch the patient is able to achieve and also to recognize his optimum pitch and establish the starting level for subsequent home and clinical practice.

2 Once the patient's pitch range is established, 'gliding' exercises that cover the full range can be introduced. These 'gliding' exercises are the forerunners of inflection and prosody work.

Using a vowel sound (eg. /a:/ or /u:/), ask the patient to glide up or down as follows:

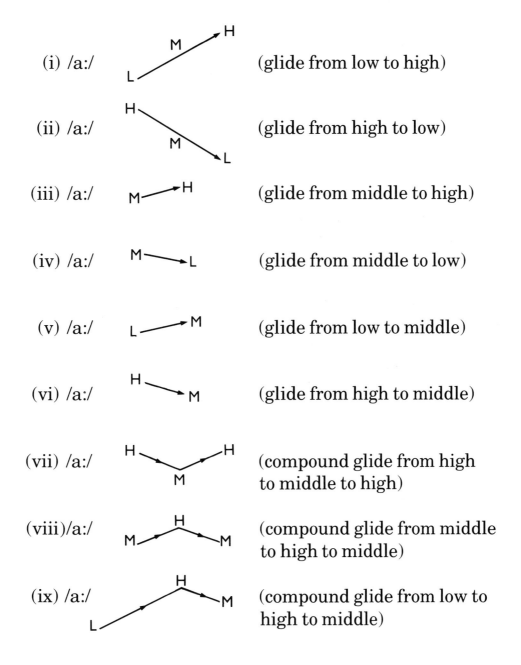

(i) /a:/   (glide from low to high)

(ii) /a:/   (glide from high to low)

(iii) /a:/   (glide from middle to high)

(iv) /a:/   (glide from middle to low)

(v) /a:/   (glide from low to middle)

(vi) /a:/   (glide from high to middle)

(vii) /a:/   (compound glide from high to middle to high)

(viii)/a:/   (compound glide from middle to high to middle)

(ix) /a:/   (compound glide from low to high to middle)

As the patient listens, then imitates these different inflection patterns, it should become clear that these variations may indicate changes in the meaning or the mood expressed. A rising inflection may indicate surprise, excitement or anticipation; whilst a falling inflection may indicate sadness, boredom or disappointment. Compound inflections may indicate a double meaning or sarcasm.

3 More subtle changes of inflection may be introduced by extending the use of the CV structure and by asking the patient to imitate the therapist in the following exercises.

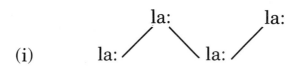

(i)

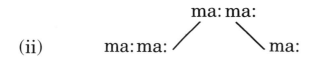

(ii)

(iii)

(iv)

The above can be extended into a definite prosody exercise by substituting words for the CV syllables, so that it becomes evident where, in normal speech, variation of inflection or intonation is required.

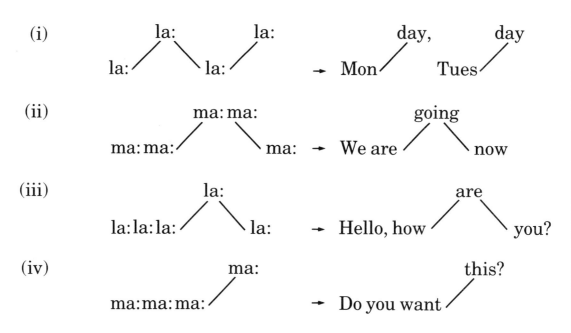

(i)

(ii)

(iii)

(iv)

This task can be made as complex as the therapist feels necessary. If the patient is coping well, it is probably appropriate to move into a more contextual framework and introduce a number of examples from everyday speech, newspaper and magazine articles, plays, poetry, etc. (For further exercise material see the reading passages in Chapter 9, page 59.)

Resonance

'Hypernasality is an excessively undesirable amount of perceived nasal cavity resonance during the phonation of vowels.' (Boone, 1983) This is a common feature of some types of dysarthria and is usually due to weakness and/or inco-ordination of the soft palate and/or palato-pharyngeal muscles.

Another type of nasal resonance problem is described by Boone as 'assimilative nasality', defined as the nasality which occurs in vowels adjacent to the three nasal consonants. 'It would appear that the velopharyngeal port is opened too soon and remains open too long, so that vowel resonance preceding and following nasal consonant resonance is also nasalised.' This sluggishness and inco-ordination of the velopharyngeal muscles may also be a feature of dysarthria.

Boone states that 'there is probably no area of voice therapy more neglected or more confusing than therapy for nasal resonance problems'. The most usual cause of hypernasality in dysarthria is incompetent or sluggish palato-pharyngeal valving; but it may also be a result of faulty tongue positioning arising from weakness or inco-ordination of tongue movements. There are, therefore, several approaches to the treatment of hypernasality.

Surgical intervention involving the construction of a pharyngeal flap is probably the most extreme form of treatment. (For further information readers are referred to Chapter 7, Surgical and prosthetic management of neurogenic speech disorders, in *Clinical management of neurogenic communication disorders,* Ed. Johns, 1978). It is more likely, however, that a prosthesis may be fitted—the so-called palatal lift—which 'typically consists of a palatal portion with hooks that attach to the patient's teeth and a posterior extension that elevates the soft palate to the posterior pharyngeal wall, thereby producing a mechanical obstruction between the oral and nasal cavities' (Rosenbek and La Pointe, 1978).

A more temporary palatal training device may be used during therapy sessions. This device is connected to a visual display which provides feedback to the patient when palatal movement is achieved. Where nasal emission is a problem then the See scope, an instrument for detecting nasal emission (CC Publications 1985), may be useful. This also provides visual feedback to the patient. The age-old piece of cotton wool or paper on a flat surface, or a metal mirror which will fog in the presence of airflow, continue to be useful visual feedback devices. The above-mentioned training devices may be used in conjunction with the more conventional methods of therapy for hypernasality.

It is important, firstly, to establish whether there is a gag reflex present. This is very relevant where there are feeding and swallowing problems. The establishing of a gag reflex is also important in relation to phonation. PNF techniques, as described by Langley and Darvill (1979), may be found useful. To stimulate the reflex, gently and slowly 'walk' a cotton wool bud or spatula along the surface of the tongue from the front towards the back or along the hard palate from the alveolar ridge towards the soft palate.

Strengthening the soft palate and encouraging sustained velopharyngeal closure are the main aims in therapy.

Exercises

Resonance

1 Encourage the patient to take a deep breath, then hold his lips together and blow out his cheeks, holding this position for a few seconds before releasing the breath. (Pinch the nares if this will help prevent nasal emission.)

2 Blowing exercises may be useful – and the use of straws of different bore-diameters will also assist lip closure and strength.

To facilitate the co-ordination of the palato-pharyngeal movement required during speech, it is important to progress to speech sound practice.

3 Practise oral plosives – labial, alveolar then velar – followed by a vowel sound (eg. /ba: da: ga:/)

4 Practise oral fricatives followed by a vowel, eg. /fa: sa: ʃa:/

5 Practise alternating oral and nasal consonants in nonsense syllables and monosyllabic words.

    eg.   (i) /ba: ma ; ma: ba:/

           (ii) me, pea ; me, bee

                my, pie ; my, buy

                no, so ; might, sight

6 Practise clusters containing oral and nasal sounds in syllables and words.

    eg.   (i) /sma: smi: snəʊ: snei/

           (ii) smile, smack

                smart, smooth

                snap, snip

                snort, snail.

CHAPTER 8

MOVEMENT OF FACIAL MUSCULATURE AND DIADOCHOKINETIC RATES

'Great precision of timing and strength of contraction, range of movement, speed of movement, and accuracy of movement direction are required for the proper production of speech. Impairment of these neuro-muscular events by neurologic disease affects all aspects of motor speech.' (Darley, Aronson and Brown, 1975)

Although this statement applies to all aspects of motor speech, including respiration, phonation, resonance, articulation and prosody, it is perhaps most obviously applicable to articulation and the articulatory musculature since this is often an important focus of dysarthria therapy.

Articulation requires normal function of the jaws, lips, tongue and palate. Abnormality of function of any of these can disrupt the speech signal. For example, facial and/or lip weakness may affect /p/; /b/; /m/; while weakness or limited movement of the tongue may directly affect the production of /l/; /s/; /t/, etc. While the focal point of much dysarthria therapy will be articulation, it is the considered opinion of many authorities, such as Darley, Aronson and Brown (1975), Rosenbek and La Pointe (1978), and the strong conviction of the authors, that much exercise and facilitation of movement of the articulators is a prerequisite of accurate articulation, and hence improved intelligibility.

In Chapter 2 a summary is given of the salient features of neuro-muscular functioning as described in great detail in *Motor Speech Disorders* (Darley, Aronson and Brown, 1975). These six properties are strength of muscular contraction, the speed of movement, the range of excursion of the part being moved, accuracy of movement, steadiness of contraction and the muscular tone.

This chapter seeks to provide a programme of therapy to facilitate these aspects of neuro-muscular function with particular attention to the strength, range, accuracy and speed of movement. Chapter 9 will seek to incorporate this increased precision of muscular movement into a programme to improve specific articulation. The two chapters, therefore, should be considered as having the same aim, namely to facilitate movement of the articulators and hence improve articulation.

Proprioceptive Neuro–muscular Facilitation (P.N.F.)

'The principles behind the restoration of function are similar in the face, tongue and throat to those which govern restoration of function in, for example, the upper extremity' (de Jersey, 1975).

An understanding of this fact has led speech therapists in recent years to use some of the P.N.F. techniques known to physiotherapy colleagues since they were developed by Kabat and Knott between 1943 and 1951, and to apply these to the speech and respiratory musculature.

Readers are referred to the excellent booklet produced by Judith Langley and Gill Darvill in 1979 *P.N.F.—A Practical Manual* for specific guidance in the use and application of P.N.F. and other techniques in the treatment of adult dysarthic and dyspraxic patients. In this chapter an outline only will be given of some of the key concepts of P.N.F. as described mainly by Langley and Darvill, but also by Rowe (1975), Knott (1954), Rosenbek and La Pointe (1978).

Facilitation refers to 'increasing the excitability of a neurone by bombarding it with impulses' (Knott, 1954). This facilitation may be achieved by two methods, which are often used in conjunction with each other. These are *stimulation* and *manipulation*.

'(a) *Stimulation* may be by *icing* or *brushing*.

(i) *Icing*
The principle is to ice the area of the face which is immediately above the muscle and/or supplied by the same cranial nerve. Icing facilitates movement instantaneously but its effects do not last, so exercise should be done immediately. Apply ice, using cubes or crushed ice in a disposable surgical glove or the corner of a polythene bag.
(CAUTION: Excessive icing causes 'burns' and will actually inhibit the desired movement. Five seconds icing is sufficient.)

(ii) *Brushing*
Unlike icing, optimum results of brushing occur after a time-lag of twenty/thirty minutes.
Hand brushing: A soft but firm camel hair or other medium sized paintbrush is held in the hand in a 'pencil grip'. Light, rapid stroking along the muscle belly for the duration of one minute (eg. on soft palate or around the margin of the lips) should be followed by activity.
(CAUTION: Certain patients may be hypersensitive to such stimulation. Gradual desensitization of the whole region may be necessary in these cases.)

(b) *Manipulation* may be by *pressure, stretch* and/or *resistance*.
Facial muscles tend not to move in isolation

but in groups or 'patterns of movement' (this can be demonstrated graphically by asking someone to 'wrinkle your nose' and noting how many parts of the face become involved when procerus is activated in this way). So work on both sides of the face at once, even if this means applying greater resistance to the unaffected side whilst assisting the corresponding muscles on the weak side.

(i) *Pressure:* is applied by finger or thumb tips (eg. stroking pressure applied to the extrinsic tongue muscles under the chin and static pressure applied to the hyoid bone, both used to assist swallowing).

(ii) *Stretch:* is achieved by repeated small stretches applied with the finger tips to the contracting muscle fibres during a movement, to stimulate greater contraction (eg. outward 'flicking' along the contracting risorius muscles to facilitate smiling).

Stretch and pressure may be used to facilitate a movement of which the patient is not yet capable without help. Treatment will often, therefore, start with these and progress to the application of resistance.

(iii) *Resistance* in this context is the application of pressure *in opposition* to the movement required in order to strengthen that movement. It is used only where the patient is capable to some degree of unassisted movement of the relevant muscles and is applied manually to the 'good' side, while only measured resistance is given to the weaker side.'

(Langley and Darvill, 1979)

'For muscle strengthening we rely on isotonic and isometric exercises. *Isotonic* exercises are repetitive movements without resistance and are especially useful in early sessions with severely involved patients, when the clinician is glad to be able to elicit any movement, no matter how limited in range and force. *Isometric* exercises are movements against resistance; for example, the patient opens his mouth while the clinician applies upward pressure against the bottom of the jaw. The goal is increased strength, resulting from overcoming systematically increased resistance.'

(Rosenbek and La Pointe, 1978)

In their practical manual, Langley and Darvill outline a range of exercises using these facilitatory techniques, particularly in relation to the soft palate, jaw, lips and tongue. They also suggest P.N.F. techniques to facilitate respiration, phonation and upper facial movement.

Barton Rowe (1975), in his article relating to the treatment of facial paralysis by P.N.F., underlines the sound neurophysiological basis of P.N.F. He also indicates that it has been shown that proprioceptive stimuli actually decrease fatigue, so this reinforces the appropriateness of these techniques even where there is considerable weakness of muscle groups.

Specific Exercises for Articulatory Muscles

The use of traditional exercises is particularly recommended both to supplement P.N.F. where this is practised and also to provide the patient with a programme of routine exercises which he can carry out during and between clinical sessions.

Analysis of the patient's performance in Section III of the Dysarthria Profile (movement of facial musculature) will have given the therapist an insight into the strength, range and accuracy of movement of the articulatory musculature. Section IV extends the therapist's awareness of the speed of movement of the articulators by testing the patient's diadochokinetic rates. From this information the therapist will be able to assess which muscle groups require most attention and exercise. A selection should therefore be made from the following exercises, first concentrating on the strength, range and accuracy of movement and later rehearsing the rapid, repetitive, alternating movements which are so important for the production of accurate, intelligible articulation.

Jaw

Movement goals—Depression
Elevation
Protrusion

1. Instruct the patient to lower his jaw as far as possible, and then to raise it to close his mouth. Repeat this slowly five times, then rest. (Continue to repeat this exercise in series of fives and gradually encourage the patient to increase the speed but retain the maximum excursion of movement.)

2. Instruct the patient to protrude his lower jaw and move it *gently* from side to side. Repeat slowly five times, then rest. Continue this exercise with the suggestion to make it into an exaggerated, rotating, chewing movement with (a) the mouth closed and (b) the mouth open.

Lips

Movement goals—Lip rounding
Lip spreading
Lip closing
Lip opening

1. Instruct the patient to push his lips forwards as far as possible (into the position for /u:/) and then pull back as far as possible (into the position for /i:/). Repeat five times slowly, then rest. Continue this exercise, gradually building up the number of repetitions between each rest. Gradually increase the speed of these alternating movements, retaining the maximum excursion of movement.

2. Instruct the patient to pull up and back one corner of the mouth, hold it, and then return to rest. Repeat five times, then rest.

Repeat this exercise, pulling back the opposite corner of the mouth, and then return to rest. Repeat five times, then rest.

3. To strengthen lip closure, ask the patient to hold a tongue guide between closed lips. (Rosenbek, 1978, suggests a plastic lip-shaped device with a string fastened to it to allow the clinician to pull against the device while the patient tries to hold it between his lips. Froeschells, cited by Rosenbek, 1978, recommends different-sized corks, beginning with small ones and graduating to larger ones as strength is increased.)

This exercise may be varied in several ways:

(i) Encourage the patient to hold the object between his lips for increasing lengths of time—indicated by the clinician counting aloud or by use of a stop watch.

(ii) Encourage the patient to hold the object firmly between his lips while the therapist tries to pull it away. The tongue guide may be used lengthways along the whole length of the lips or with its thin end held centrally between the lips.

4. Instruct the patient to hold his lips together and blow out his cheeks (the space between lips and gums should also fill with air). The patient should hold this position for a few seconds and then expel the air suddenly (to aid this plosion, the patient may be instructed to push his cheeks with the fingers of both hands). Repeat this exercise an increasing number of times.

5. Instruct the patient to open his mouth wide and then alter his lip position by alternately pushing his lips forwards and stretching them back (moving from the position for /ɔ:/ to the position for /ɑ:/). Repeat five times, then rest. Continue this exercise, increasing both the number and the rate of repetitions, but maintaining the full range of movement.

Tongue

Movement goals—Protrusion
Retraction
Elevation of tip
Elevation of blade
Lateral movement
Circular movement

1. Ask the patient to protrude his tongue as far as possible and then retract and roll it backwards in the mouth. Repeat five times and then rest. Continue this exercise, gradually increasing the number of tongue movements between each rest.

(i) To encourage full protrusion of the tongue, the therapist may hold a tongue guide in front of the patient's lips for him to touch with the tongue tip.

(ii) To strengthen the tongue in protrusion, systematic resistance may be applied by pushing against the tongue tip with the spatula.

(iii) To increase the rate of movement, encourage the patient to increase the number of repetitions while retaining the full range of movement. (A stop watch and digital counter may be used to monitor the rate and number of repetitions.)

2. Ask the patient to raise his tongue tip both (i) inside the mouth—to the alveolar ridge, and (ii) outside the mouth—beyond the upper lip. Repeat this up and down movement five times and then rest. Continue this exercise, gradually increasing the number of tongue movements between each rest. (It may be necessary to hold the chin so that the mouth remains open throughout the exercise and the lower jaw does not assist the elevation of the tongue.)

(i) The tongue guide may be used to assist and then resist elevation and depression of the tongue tip in order to strengthen this particular movement.

(ii) Encourage increasing rate of elevation/depression of tongue tip inside the mouth and monitor as in the previous exercise.

3. Ask the patient to elevate the blade of his tongue to the hard palate. The tongue guide may be used to indicate the target point of contact. The movement may also be facilitated if the tongue tip remains in firm contact behind the lower teeth. Repeat five times and

then rest. Continue the exercise, gradually increasing the number of movements between each rest.

4. Ask the patient to move his tongue tip from one corner of the mouth to the other. Repeat this exercise five times and then rest. Continue the exercise gradually increasing the number of complete movements between rests.

(i) The tongue guide may be used again to assist and then resist the lateral movements. The patient should be encouraged to push against the tongue guide placed along the margin of the tongue. In the case of unilateral weakness, the tongue guide should be placed along the margin of the stronger side and resistance should be gradually increased.

(ii) Encourage increasing rate of lateral tongue movements and monitor as in the previous exercises.

5. Lateral movement of the tongue may also be facilitated by asking the patient to push out each cheek in turn with the tongue tip.

6. The range of tongue movements normally used during eating and to aid oral hygiene should also be practised.

(i) Move the tongue tip between the teeth and lips and 'sweep' across from one side to the other over the upper teeth and return to the other side over the lower teeth ('cleaning teeth' movement).

(ii) Move the tongue tip up and down against the inside of each cheek in a 'sweeping' movement.

Soft Palate

Movement goal—Elevation

'Inconsistent or consistent hypernasality is the most frequently reported resonance abnormality in the dysarthrias.' (Rosenbek and La Pointe, 1978.)

This is often attributable to the weakness of the soft palate or to the lack of co-ordination and/or reduced range or speed of movement of the palate. It is particularly difficult to remediate the soft palate and a number of clinicians and researchers have recommended a range of prosthetic devices to aid elevation of the palate. These palatal lift prostheses are discussed by Rosenbek and La Pointe (1978), Shaughnessy, Netsell and Farrage (1983) and others. While some writers report good success rates, others remain guarded in their evaluation of the efficacy of such devices. Rosenbek, in particular, points out that 'neither the patient nor the clinician should expect more of the prosthesis than the patient's symptom complex will allow'. On the more positive side, he also comments that 'often competence with the lift will evolve slowly as the patient works to improve his articulation, modify his rate, and so on.'
Langley and Darvill (1979) advocate the application of ice, on a cotton bud, to the unaffected side of the velum, using an upward stroking movement. Occasionally, also, surgical intervention has been used to aid velopharyngeal closure in the form of an injection of Teflon along Passavant's line.
It is difficult to exercise the soft palate without introducing voicing and articulation of specific phenome combinations.

1. Encouraging the patient to initiate a yawn may facilitate elevation of the palate.

2. Ask the patient to repeat a series of /aː/ sounds—encourage a definite 'attack' on phonation to facilitate the elevation.

3. (i) Introduce the repetition of a series of plosive and open vowel sounds: eg./paː paː paː/; /daː daː daː/

    (ii) Proceed to a series of fricatives and closed vowel sounds: eg /siː siː siː/; /ʃuː ʃuː ʃuː/

    (iii) Repeat a series of nasal and voiced plosive and vowel sounds: eg. /mbaː mbaː mbaː/; /ndaː ndaː ndaː/; /ŋgaː ŋgaː ŋgaː/

    (iv) Repeat a series of fricative and nasal and vowel sounds: eg. /smaː smaː smaː/; /sniː sniː sniː/

Diadochokinesis

Many of the exercises described in this chapter have introduced the concept of increasing the rate of repetitive movements. The speed of movement of the articulators has an important bearing on the precision of articulation and the intelligibility of speech. The profile described in Chapter 4 illustrates the impoverished diadochokinetic rate of the patient with a flaccid dysarthria. This was a major contributory factor in his poor articulation and greatly reduced intelligibility. Diadochokinetic rate exercises should therefore form an important extension to lip and tongue exercises in particular. They should also be a major part of the early articulation work.

It is recommended that diadochokinetic exercises be attempted first without phonation (ie. movement of the articulators only) and later with phonation (ie. repetition of sequences of nonsense syllables).

1. Jaw: Alternately open and close mouth.

2. Lips: Alternately push lips forwards and stretch back.

3. Tongue:
   (i) Alternately protrude and retract tongue
   (ii) Alternately elevate and lower tip of tongue inside mouth
   (iii) Alternately move tongue from one corner of mouth to the other.

4. Repeat:
   (i) /uː iː uː iː uː iː ...../
   (ii) /daː daː daː ...../ ; /taː taː taː ...../
   (iii) /gaː gaː gaː ...../ ; /kaː kaː kaː ...../
   (iv) /baː baː baː ...../ ; /paː paː paː ...../
   (v) /kaː laː kaː laː ...../ ; /laː kaː laː kaː ...../
   (vi) /tə kə tə kə ...../ ; /kə tə kə tə ...../
   (vii) /p t k p t k ...../ ; /b d g b d g ...../

Repeat each of these exercises as rapidly as possible: either specify a number of repetitions (perhaps 10) to be attempted as fast as possible, or alternatively indicate the number of seconds the patient should aim to keep producing the sounds (perhaps five seconds).

CHAPTER 9
ARTICULATION

'The prime target for the remedial programme of most dysarthric patients probably will be articulation' (Darley, Aronson and Brown, 1975).

The majority of dysarthric patients present with articulatory difficulties which contribute to their lack of intelligibility. The starting point for articulation therapy may be one of two apparently opposite poles. If, on assessment, the patient is noted to be able to articulate most sounds correctly in isolation or in simple, monosyllabic words, but in continuous speech or polysyllabic words his articulation breaks down, then this would suggest the need for a therapeutic approach based on controlling the rate of his speech. On the other hand, if the patient has problems with the production of sounds in isolation, then this would suggest that a systematic approach is required, working on individual sounds before proceeding to various sound combinations and then to single words and phrases.

A. Allowing more time for Articulation

Some groups of dysarthric patients (eg. those with Parkinson's Disease) are able to produce all the sounds of speech in isolation, indicating more or less adequate range, accuracy and speed of movement of the articulators. However, in such cases articulatory precision may be lost when the patient attempts longer words, phrases or conversational speech. The following suggestions for therapy may be helpful.

Encourage the patient to slow down his rate of speaking in reading and in conversation. This will allow him more time to complete the articulatory movements required for each sound (see exercises, page 42).

To aid the control of speed and hence articulation in continuous speech, give the patient a short passage of prose to read aloud. The passage should be clearly marked out in phrases and the patient must be given specific instructions to read to the bar line and then stop, breathe if necessary, then read to the next bar line. It may be necessary to cover up most of the script with a sheet of paper to reveal one line of prose only at a time. The choice of a prose passage will depend upon its relevance and interest to the individual, and also on the patient's pre-morbid reading ability. See exercise on page 43.

To facilitate the control of speed of articulation in spontaneous conversational speech, engage in a short question-and-answer session with the patient. The questions should be structured so that the patient's answers can be short, simple phrases which he can control for speed, whilst at the same time concentrating on clear articulation.

eg. Therapist: What is your name?

Patient: John Smith

Therapist: What's your favourite food?

Patient: Fish and chips.

Therapist: What T.V. programme do you like to watch?

Patient: Coronation Street.

In all the above exercises in which the patient demonstrates his potential to achieve clear speech, it is vital that he should be encouraged to:

(i) reduce the speed

(ii) shorten phrasing

(iii) use syllable-timed speech if necessary

In addition to these he should:

(iv) exaggerate articulatory movements and 'over-articulate' medial and final consonants (eg. baKing; gaTe)

(v) take time when articulating complicated consonant clusters (eg. s.w i f.t.l y; p.r es.c.r.i p.tion)

B. Systematic Phonetic Approach

Where the patient has specific difficulty producing individual phonemes or moving from one phoneme to the next, the therapist must first ensure that a considerable amount of pre-speech work has been carried out. This includes exercising the articulatory muscles and practising diadochokinetic rates (see Chapter 8). Only when the neuro-muscular aspects of range, strength, co-ordination, accuracy and speed of movement of the tongue, lips, jaw and palate have been dealt with at some length, should the therapist proceed to specific articulation work.

The steps in therapy are similar to those in any systematic articulation programme. The choice of which phoneme to begin with will depend on the patient's individual problems. Generally, one should begin with the phonemes he finds easiest and proceed systematically to the more difficult ones. Phonemes that are easily 'seen' such as bilabials, are often the best ones to begin with.

A procedure for work on /b/ is suggested below. A similar approach can be employed to facilitate production of other problem sounds:

1. Practise /b/ in isolation.

To elicit the voiced bilabial plosive, some of the following stages may be necessary:

(i) Encourage the patient to watch as the therapist produces the sound.

(ii) Encourage the patient to look in a mirror as he produces the sound.

(iii) Hold the patient's lips together and encourage him to blow out his cheeks—to build up intra-oral air pressure—and then suddenly let go his lips simultaneously as he tries to say the sound.

(iv) The P.N.F. techniques outlined in Chapter 8, concentrating on the lips and lip closure, may be attempted immediately prior to these exercises to produce the bilabial plosives.

2. Practise /b/ in final position of VC syllables /æ b/

3. Practise /b/ in final position of CVC syllables /k æ b/ (cab)

4. Practise /b/ in medial position of VCV syllables /a: ba:/

5. Practise /b/ in initial position of CV syllables /bi :/ (bee)

6. Practise /b/ in initial position of CVC syllables /b æ d/ (bad)

7. Practise /b/ in varying positions in one and two syllable words (tub, bite, cabbage)

8. Practise /b/ in varying positions in short phrases and in sentences (eg. bee-hive; a big bottle; buy a book about birds; bubble and squeak; I bought cabbage and beetroot).

9. Practise /b/ in various clusters (eg. black; bring).

10. Practise alliterative tongue twisters (eg. Betty bought a bit of bitter butter).

With adult patients it is probably best to try to use 'real' words where possible in the above exercises. However, when this is not appropriate (eg. 2 and 4 above) the patient will usually accept that this is an exercise situation involving the use of 'nonsense' words. For the therapist, at this stage the phonetic build up is more important than the reality of the words used.

When facilitating and improving the production of any problem sound, practice should proceed through the following stages:

1. words—monosyllabic and polysyllabic

2. phrases

3. sentences

4. controlled reading

5. question-and-answer exercises

6. conversational speech

Lists of words and phrases and some examples of short prose passages for reading aloud are given at the end of this chapter. Selection of these should be made with care so that they are appropriate to the individual patient, both in terms of the practice required and bearing in mind reading ability, background and interests.

Compensation Techniques

It is recognized that some patients will not be able to achieve completely accurate articulation because of weakness, restricted range or slowness of movement of the articulators. In such cases it may be necessary to teach compensatory methods of articulation. Some examples of these are listed below. These compensatory strategies will result in reasonably adequate and intelligible approximations to the sounds (*see page 43*).

Exercises

Allowing more time for articulation

1   (a) If the patient has difficulty with continuous prose then present him with a series of short, simple phrases to read slowly and clearly.

eg.
> Today is Thursday.
> I need to buy petrol.
> The kettle's boiling.
> Wash the dishes.
> Give me that newspaper.
> A cup of coffee.
> Take the dog for a walk.
> The music's too loud.
> The postman's here.
> Water the plants.

(b) If the patient is unable to control the speed in these short phrases, then it may be necessary to introduce syllable-timed speech. In this case, beat out each syllable by tapping with a pencil, to begin with, in unison with the patient. Then ask him to repeat the phrase on his own. A pacing board may also be used to control the speed.

> To – day – is – Thurs – day.
>
> I – need – to – buy – pet – rol.
>
> The – ke – ttle's – boi – ling.
>
> Wash – the – dish – es.

2   Where there is difficulty with polysyllabic words then it is important to teach a syllable-by-syllable approach, beginning with two-syllable words and gradually working towards three-, four- and five-syllable words.

eg.
car – pet ;   win – dow ;   birth – day ;
Mon – day ;   ga – rage ;   pa – per ;

news – pa – per ;   ca – len – dar ;   hos – pi – tal ;
pho – to – graph ;   Ger – man – y ;   Sat – ur – day ;

su – per – mar – ket ;   tel – e – vi – sion ;
A – me – ri ca ;   res – pon – si – ble ;

e – lec – tri – ci – ty ;   ex – am – in – a – tion ;
prin – ci – pa – li – ty ;   au – di – to – ri – um ;
pro – fess – ion – a – lly ;   in – ac – cess – i – ble.

Exercise

BIG BEN

The tallest of the three towers / that rise above / the Houses of Parliament / is often called / Big Ben. / This is really / inaccurate / because Big Ben / is the name of the bell / inside the three hundred / and twenty feet / clock tower. / This giant bell / weighs thirteen and a half tons / and was named after a man / called Sir Benjamin Hall. / From the ground / it is hard to realize / just how big / this clock really is. /

The diameter of the clock / is twenty three feet, / and each figure / is two feet high. / The hands of the clock / are also gigantic, / the small one / being nine feet tall / while the large one / stands fourteen feet in height, / twice as high / as a normal door. /

The chimes of Big Ben / are known all over the world, / as they are often heard / booming their message / over the radio. /

Compensation Techniques

Difficult Sound	Suggested Alternative
/l/ with tongue tip	raise blade of tongue, keeping tongue tip in lower position
/s/ with tongue tip raised to alveolus	produce /s/ with tongue tip immediately behind lower teeth
/p/ /b/ with lip closure	produce plosive with upper teeth making contact with lower lip (ie. produce a 'plosive' /f/ or /v/)
/m/ with lip closure	place upper teeth on lower lip and produce nasal sound
/n/ with tongue tip	raise blade of tongue, keeping tongue tip in lower position
/t/ /d/ with tongue tip	raise blade of tongue, keeping tongue tip in lower position

Exercises

1 Articulation – Word Lists

/p/

CV	VC	CVC	(C)VCV(C)	(C)CCV(C)
pea	up	peep	paper	play
paw	op	pop	puppy	plan
pie	ape	pip	pupil	plot
pay	(h)ip	pup	puppet	pram
par	(h)oop	pipe	peeping	prawn
poor	(h)ope	Pope	pepper	pray
peer	(h)arp		popping	spoon
	(h)eap		piper	spark
			pauper	speak
			purple	splay
				splash
				split
				spray
				sprawl
				sprite

/b/

CV	VC	CVC	(C)VCV(C)	(C)CCV(C)
bee	Abe	Bob	baby	blue
boy	(h)ub	babe	Bobby	black
buy	(h)ob	bib	barber	blank
bar		boob	bubble	blot
bow		barb	bobbin	brown
beer			bobbing	bring
bore			Bible	brass
				break

/t/

CV	VC	CVC	(C)VCV(C)	(C)CCV(C)
tea	at	tart	titter	tree
toy	it	tight	tatter	try
tie	art	toot	teeter	trip
two	eat	tit	totter	trap
toe	out	tout		twin
tar	(h)at	taught		twine
tear	(h)oot	teat		twist
	(h)ot	tote		sty
	(h)ut			stew
				stamp
				stop
				strap
				strike

/d/

CV	VC	CVC	(C)CVC(C)	(C)CCV(C)
day	add	dad	Dido	dry
do	odd	did	daddy	draw
dye	aid	deed	dawdle	drop
door	eyed	dead	doodle	drip
dare	owed	dud		drive
deer	(h)ard	dyed		dream
	(h)id	dared		dwell
				dwarf

/k/

CV	VC	CVC	(C)VCV(C)	(C)CCV(C)
car	ark	cake	cooker	clay
key	ache	coke	kicker	clue
core	oak	cook	cackle	clap
care	irk	kick	cocky	clock
Kay	eke	cock	cockle	clip
coy	(h)ack	cork		class
coo	(h)awk	kirk		crab
cow	(h)ike			crash
	(h)ook			cruel
				cream
				queen
				quick
				scream
				scrape
				screw

/g/

CV	VC	CVC	(C)VCV(C)	(C)CCV(C)
go	ugh	gag	gaga	glove
gay	(h)ug	gig	gurgle	glad
gear	(h)ag	dog	giggle	glee
gore	(h)og	tug	gaggle	glue
guy	(H)aigue	wig	goggle	glade
		rug		glide
		beg		grey
		keg		grow
				green
				grab
				groan
				growl

/m/

CV	VC	CVC	(C)VCV(C)	(C)CCV(C)
me	am	maim	mummy	smart
my	I'm	mime	murmur	smile
mow	aim	Ma'am	mammal	smooth
moo	ohm	mum	miming	smash
may	arm			small
ma	(h)am			smell
more	(h)im			smack
	(h)ome			

/n/

CV	VC	CVC	(C)VCV(C)	(C)CCV(C)
no	on	nine	nanny	sneer
nay	in	none	any	snow
now	an	noon	honey	snipe
nigh	earn	non	Tony	snip
knee	(h)en	noun	winner	snail
near		Nan	banner	snap
gnaw			money	snort
			canning	snarl
			gunner	

/ ŋ /

CV	VC	CVC	(C)VCV(C)	(C)CCV(C)
	(h)ang	long	hanger	linger
	(h)ung	gang	singer	longer
		wing	longing	hunger
		pang	banging	younger
		song	hanging	jungle
		ding	singing	mangle
		wrong	winging	mongrel
		tongue		

/f/

CV	VC	CVC	(C)VCV(C)	(C)CCV(C)
far	off	deaf	offer	flow
fair	if	tough	wafer	fly
four	(h)oof	cough	buffer	flee
fear	(h)alf	laugh	leafy	flew
Fay	huff	muff	fearful	flash
fur		thief	laughing	free
fire		chief	coughing	fry
fee		buff	deafen	frog
few			orphan	fruit

/v/

CV	VC	CVC	(C)VCV(C)	(C)CCV(C)
via	of	verve	viva	
vow	Ave	five	hover	
vie	(h)ave	give	hoover	
veer	(h)ive	Dave	heaving	
view	(H)ove	move	woven	
	(h)eave	cave	oval	
		love		
		weave		

/θ/

CV	VC	CVC	(C)VCV(C)	(C)CCV(C)
thigh	earth	path	Cathy	three
thaw	oath	bath	ether	thrive
Theo	(h)ath	Keith	bathing	throat
	(h)eath	Beth	Ethel	through
	(h)earth	south	anything	thrash
		north	Athens	thrall
		moth		thread
		Ruth		throb
		teeth		throw
		faith		thwack
		mouth		thwart

/ð/

CV	VC	CVC	(C)VCV(C)	(C)CCV(C)
the		bathe	father	
thee		soothe	weather	
thy		lathe	gather	
though		loath	other	
thou		with	mother	
they			heather	
there			dither	
			hither	
			teething	
			scything	
			breathing	

/s/

CV	VC	CVC	(C)VCV(C)	(C)CCV(C)
see	ass	cease	Bessy	speak
saw	ace	sauce	cissy	spare
sigh	ice	source	fussy	spot
say	(h)iss	bus	kissing	stay
Sue	(h)ouse	pass	faces	stop
so	(h)orse	loss	missing	stool
sewer		mouse	glasses	slay
sow		nurse		sleep
		nice		slope
		puss		sky
		hiss		skip
		dose		ski
				smile
				smart
				smear
				snail
				snape
				swear
				sweet
				swipe
				spray
				spree
				spring
				stray
				stroll
				strum
				squire
				squaw

/z/

CV	VC	CVC	(C)VCV(C)	(C)CCV(C)
zoo	ooze	zoos	easy	
Zoe	ease	sieze	busy	
	(h)aze	says	lazy	
	(h)ose	sews	hazy	
	(wh)ose	sighs	losing	
		fuse	boozer	
			puzzle	
			housing	

/ʃ/

CV	VC	CVC	(C)VCV(C)	(C)CCV(C)
she	ash	dish	ashes	shred
shy	(h)ush	wash	dishes	shrew
show	(h)arsh	bash	washing	shrewd
shoe		push	lotion	shriek
shore		sash	cushion	shrine
shah		rash	portion	shroud
sheer		lush	cashier	shrub
		gosh		
		quiche		

/tʃ/

CV	VC	CVC	(C)VCV(C)	(C)CCV(C)
chew	itch	church	butcher	
char	arch	batch	richer	
chair	each	witch	patching	
cheer	ouch	fetch	satchel	
chow	(h)atch	Dutch	ketchup	
	(h)itch	much	catches	
	(h)utch	rich	hatching	
		porch	fetches	
		match	touching	
		larch	watches	
		coach		

/dʒ/

CV	VC	CVC	(C)VCV(C)	(C)CCV(C)
jar	age	judge	wager	
jaw	edge	sage	badger	
jeer	(H)odge	badge	ledger	
Jew	(h)uge	Madge	ages	
joy		ledge	ridges	
gee		ridge	pages	
jay		page	ajar	
Joe		seige	dodging	
			hedging	
			forging	

/l/

CV	VC	CVC	(C)VCV(C)	(C)CCV(C)
lay	ale	lull	ally	blue
lah	all	lisle	Ely	black
low	eel	loll	lily	blow
lie	isle	pool	holy	play
law	earl	fail	follow	plight
loo	ill	ball	yellow	please
leer	owl	shall	below	glass
	(H)ull	Jill	Millie	glare
			Molly	glee
			holly	glue
			bully	clear
			calling	Claire
			falling	clue
			darling	clown
			dealer	fly
				flare
				flee
				flake
				sleep
				slam
				sly
				splay
				splash

/w/

CV	VC	CVC	(C)VCV(C)	(C)CCV(C)
why			away	swing
where			firework	swine
whirr			forward	swoop
we			earwig	swap
war				switch
way				swim
woe				twin
woo				twine
				thwart
				dwarf
				queen
				quail
				choir
				squeeze
				squirrel

/r/

CV	VC	CVC	(C)VCV(C)	(C)CCV(C)
ray			arrow	fry
roe			airy	free
raw			eerie	Fred
Roy			fury	prize
row			dowry	pray
rare			barrow	prim
rye			marrow	brown
			carry	brave
			error	breeze
			berry	cry
			orange	crawl
			marriage	crave
			carrot	crew
			syrup	grow
			Cyril	great
				growl
				through
				three
				throat
				dry
				drop
				try
				tray
				shrub
				shrine
				screw
				scream
				scrap
				string
				stray
				street
				spring
				sprawl
				spruce

/j/

CV	*VC*	*CVC*	*(C)VCV(C)*	*(C)CCV(C)*
ye				
you				
your				
yea				
year				

/ʒ/

CV	*VC*	*CVC*	*(C)VCV(C)*	*(C)CCV(C)*
		beige	azure	
			leisure	
			measure	
			fusion	
			seizure	
			closure	

II Alliterative Phrases for Articulation Practice

A selection of the following may be helpful for home practice.

1. Bilabials

A big blue badly bleeding blister.

Betty bought a bit of butter.

Buy Bridge's British breeches.

Peter Piper picked a peck of pickled pepper.

A pale pink proud peacock pompously preened its pretty plumage.

Please Paul pause for applause.

Many million mini-Minors milling round Manchester.

My maths master munches marmalade muffins.

Merry moments make Madge mischievous.

2. Alveolars

A sick sparrow sang six sad Spring songs.

Down the slippery slope they slipped sitting slightly sideways.

Seventeen slimy slugs sat on the sand.

Sixty-six slick soldiers.

Tying tapes takes time.

A twin-track tape recorder.

The twenty-to-two train to Tooting tooted through the tunnel.

Do drop in at Dewdrop Inn.

A dozen damask dinner napkins.

Dashing Daniel danced dangerously down past Dora.

Red leather, yellow leather.

Red rubies round the ring.

Rupert wrestled rashly with Robin.

Round the rugged rocks the ragged rascal ran.

Lots of little London lamplighters.

Lame lambs limp.

Lucy lingered looking longingly for her little lass.

Nina needs nine knitting needles.

Nice nurses need necklaces.

Nine nimble noblemen nibbling nettles.

3. Velars

A cup of creamy custard cooked for Cuthbert.

Cross-eyed Clare's crazy over crosswords.

The crime completed, the criminal crawled cautiously coastward.

Granny's grey goose gobbled the grain.

Greengages grow in Gloria's garden.

Grace's grey gloves glided to the ground.

4. Dentals

They thanked them thoroughly.

They threw three thick things.

Thelma saw thistles in the thick thatch.

There are thirty thousand feathers on that thrush's throat.

We'll weather the weather whatever the weather, whether we like it or not.

5. Labio Dentals

Forty fat French frogs.

A flea and a fly got lost in a flue.

Four famished fishermen frying flying fish.

Philip forced Frank to fence.

Vera valued the various vases.

Victor viewed the vast vacant vista.

Valiant vassals vexed Victoria.

6. Palatals

Shy Sheila sat shivering in her shiny silk shirt.

Shocking shoppers shopping in Shrewsbury.

All ship shape in the fish and chip shop.

Chimes challenged the changing year.

Cheerful children chant charming tunes.

Fish and chip shop chips are soft chips.

Jean, Joan, George and Gerald judged the junior jumping.

James just jostled Jean.

Jack Jones jumped on Jimmy last June.

III Short Prose Passages for Reading Aloud

The following reading passages are marked in a variety of ways so that the therapist may select a method of assisting the patient's monitoring and control eg. to assist breathing as in passage (a). These are suggestions only – the needs of individual patients will vary considerably.

Alternatively, the therapist may simply ask the patient to read the passage aloud as general practice for accurate articulation.

In addition to reading passages, the patient may be encouraged to:

1. choose his own extract from a book or magazine to read aloud

2. write a letter and read it aloud

3. write an account of something (eg. an outing or TV programme) and read it aloud.

Passage a

[Bar lines indicate phrasing – to assist control of breathing and encourage frequent pausing.]

A DISAPPOINTED MAN

On November 25th, / 1910, / Captain Scott / had set sail / from New Zealand / in his ship / 'Terra Nova' / in a quest / to reach the South Pole. / He planted a flag / at the South Pole / on January / 17th, / 1912. / Scott had achieved / his ambition / to reach the Pole, / but he was / disappointed. / Scott had found / a small tent / and a Norwegian flag / at the Pole, / along with a note / dated December / 14th, / 1911, / wishing him / a safe return. / Captain Amundsen, / who had set out / for the Pole / at about the same time / as Scott, / but on a different route, / had arrived first. /

Passage b

[Bar lines indicate longer phrases than in (a) above.]

'HERE IS THE WEATHER FORECAST'

Everyone must have heard these words / over the radio, / and perhaps listened for a few minutes / to hear what the weather might be the next day, / but very few people realize / how much work is put into a forecast. / Meteorologists / often live for two years or more / in the frozen and bitter climate / of the Arctic wastes, / so that they can send information / about the weather. / This information / along with details from ships at sea, / planes high in the air, / and even satellites in space, / is all considered / before a weather forecast is given. / All these observations and details / must be taken at 9.00am / Greenwich Mean Time, / and then are sent via wireless, / telegraph, / telephone and radio / to a central office. /

Passage c

[—— These lines indicate the strongly stressed words and syllables.]

A FAMOUS MEETING

David Livingstone was a very famous missionary and explorer. He was a qualified doctor and worked for the London Missionary Society in Africa. Livingstone had become famous for his work in Africa, but nobody had heard of him for four and a half years and many people assumed he must have been killed. A man called Stanley was sent by an American newspaper to look for Livingstone. Stanley spent months in his search, but he finally found Livingstone, who was then nearly sixty years old. Stanley was lost for words when they met, so he just said 'Doctor Livingstone I presume?' Livingstone raised his cap and said 'Yes'.

Passage d

[The final consonants are underlined and should be read with special care.]

THE SYDNEY HARBOUR BRIDGE

The bridge that spans the entrance to Sydney Harbour in Australia has the longest steel arch in the world. It is 1650 feet (503 metres) long. This does not mean that it is the longest bridge in the world, only the longest of this type.

In this type of bridge, the weight of the traffic is supported by the arch, from which the roadway is suspended. After the approach roads have been made, the arch is then built, starting from each bank and meeting in the middle. Only when the arch is complete, is the roadway (called the deck) suspended from it.

The Sydney Harbour Bridge deck carries eight lanes of traffic, two railway lines, a bicycle track and a footway for pedestrians.

Passage e

[The consonant clusters are underlined and should be produced accurately.]

A DRASTIC CURE!

When Sir Walter Raleigh returned from an expedition to Virginia, he brought back some tobacco and became the first man in this country to start smoking. One of his faithful servants who saw smoke rising from his master's chair quickly threw a bucket of water over him to try to put out the fire. Raleigh must have been annoyed when he explained that he was not on fire, but just smoking his clay pipe of tobacco.

Nowadays, thousands of people have take up this expensive habit, and it is thought that by doing so they might be endangering their health. Perhaps it is a pity that the servant's drastic cure nearly four hundred years ago did not work.

Passage f

[The polysyllabic words are underlined and should be read with particular care.]

ZERO!

Since October 4th, 1957, when the Russians launched the first earth satellite, many rockets have thundered into the heavens. Months, sometimes years of preparation go into a rocket before it is launched, and when the word 'Zero' is given all the designers and scientists must watch with fear and excitement gripping their hearts. The rocket moves slowly at first, then gathers speed and disappears into the sky, bound for the moon. The rocket will take three to four days to travel the two-hundred and fifty thousand miles. The astronaut in his capsule will have many strange experiences. He will find himself able to float, but unable to pour liquid into a container and unable to drop anything.

CHAPTER 10
INTELLIGIBILITY AND RATE

Intelligibility

'Reduced intelligibility is a frequent, if not a universal, consequence of dysarthric speech, regardless of the underlying neuromotor deficit.' This statement by Yorkston and Beukelman (1981) appears in the introduction to their *Assessment of Intelligibility of Dysarthric Speech*. It underlines their conviction that 'intelligibility may serve as an overall index of severity', since, 'few measures, other than intelligibility of connected speech, allow the clinician to evaluate the sum of the interacting processes that are involved in speech production'.

Intelligibility is not only the index by which the dysarthric's speech will be judged, but it also indicates the overall integration and co-ordination of all of the other motor speech processes (particularly respiration, phonation and articulation). With regard to the processes listed, intelligibility is a direct result of their efficiency, but it is also inextricably linked with the suprasegmental features of rhythm, stress and intonation (*see Chapter 11*). The control of the rate of utterance is also an integral part of intelligible speech and, as such, it will be considered below in conjunction with intelligibility.

For the patient to be intelligible is the ultimate aim of all of the therapy thus far described. In the strategies outlined in the previous chapter on articulation, it is implicit that intelligibility is the primary objective of all of the phoneme, syllable, word, phrase and continuous speech practice.

Several authors have indicated that exaggerated articulatory movement is one of the keys to intelligible speech. Exercises which focus directly on movement of the articulators have been suggested in Chapter 9. However, in order to concentrate more on the carry-over of efficient articulation into continuous functional speech, some further exercises are recommended. The following activities are graded in complexity.

1. Ask the patient to repeat and/or read aloud lists of words which, in the first instance, contain some of the target sounds. The lists given in Chapter 9 may be used. Further lists, given on pages 66-69, may be used in a more random way, the object being to make each word intelligible to the listener—in this case the therapist.

In order to encourage whole-message communication, the patient may be asked to read the words out at random from the list. The therapist, meanwhile, may or may not have access to the printed list and will either write down or repeat aloud what she hears. This will help to reinforce the need for clarity and accuracy.

2. Ask the patient to repeat and/or read aloud phrases of increasing length and articulatory complexity. The aim again is for intelligibility; the method of dictating to

the therapist, as previously described, may also be used. See pages 70–72 for examples.

3. In Chapter 9 examples of fairly short, simple reading passages were given. These can be used within the context of achieving intelligible speech as well as for controlled articulation practice. To progress from this stage, a few examples of short extracts from newspapers, magazines, travel brochures, recipe books and catalogues are given on page 73. The therapist may wish to record the patient reading these and then allow him to listen to them later and discuss the level of intelligibility. On the other hand, the therapist may choose to take notes as she listens to him reading the passage, then feed back the information to the patient for verification.

4. Question-and-answer sessions may also be used to encourage intelligibility; the patient either answers the questions asked by the therapist, or role plays the quizmaster or interviewer and asks the questions of the therapist.

(i) Interview-type questions:

What is your full name?

Where do you live?

What family do you have?

Tell me about your job.

What are your hobbies/interests?

What T.V. programmes do you watch?

What do you think about the cost of petrol?

(ii) Quizzes may cover a wide range of topics and there are many quiz books available that are suitable for use in such sessions. Initially, however, it may be necessary to devise questions which the patient can answer without too much difficulty— at all times the goal must be intelligible speech.

5. There are a range of speaking situations that can provide opportunities to concentrate on intelligibility. As the patient is progressing in the use of functional, continuous speech, a selection of the following activities may be useful:

(i) describing a composite picture
(eg. from a magazine; newspaper; book)

(ii) describing a sequence of pictures which build up into a complete story
(eg. cartoon strips; visual sequencing pictures)

(iii) describing a step-by-step method
(eg. making a cup of tea; boiling an egg; changing a wheel; decorating a room)

(iv) play reading of short dialogues

(v) delivering short, prepared talks on various topics (eg. travel; holidays; the family; a day's work; buying a house; keeping a pet)

(vi) giving instructions on a particular topic which the therapist must understand and carry out (eg. peeling a potato; wiring a plug; writing a letter)

(vii) going on assignments to make a purchase or find out some specific information within the hospital (eg. from canteen; hospital shop; reception desk)

(viii) going on assignments outside the clinic (eg. to the shops; station; library; travel agent)

6. One of the most difficult tasks to test the intelligibility of a patient's speech is use of the telephone. If he has achieved intelligibility in the face-to-face situation, then a useful exercise is to practise using the telephone in a hierarchically structured way. Some examples are listed below:

(i) making internal calls from one room to another within the clinic

(ii) phoning the patient at home

(iii) asking the patient to phone the therapist from home

(iv) asking the patient to make a phone call for specific information (eg. to a cinema to ask the price of tickets or the times of performances; to the station to ask the times of train arrivals and departures)

Rate

Intrinsic to the achieving of intelligible speech is the control of the rate of speech. Yorkston and Beukelman (1981) considered rate and intelligibility to be so interlinked that the report of their own therapy programmes stated: 'control of speaking rate as a means of maximising speech intelligibility was an early goal for all subjects'.

All the above exercises in this chapter may, therefore, also be used to focus specific attention on the correct rate.

Basically, faulty speech rate implies one of three options: excessive speed, insufficient speed, or the gradual increase of speed during the course of an utterance. The latter is known as festinance.

Slow Rate

On the whole, the rate of speech is usually slow if the patient has difficulty in co-ordinating the motor speech musculature at the normal rate. In this case, it is often better to allow the patient to keep to a slower rate, since to try to speed up might interfere with the intelligibility and the accuracy of articulation. Only gradually should the patient be encouraged to try to speed up his speech a little, within phrases, using the pauses to rest and replenish the breath.

Fast, and Festinant speech

There are several ways of reducing the overall rate of speech or of helping the patient to maintain an appropriate rate throughout speech.

1. Yorkston and Beukelman (1981) suggest that there should be 'rigid imposition of rate'. In this system the patient is required to point to the first letter of each word on an alphabet board as he speaks that word. This not only slows a speaker's rate, but it also gives the communication partner extra information in the form of the initial letter of each word.

2. Another technique for imposing rate control is the pacing board described by Helm (1979). The board may be of a simple construction such as a piece of wood the length of a ruler with raised divisions at 1″ intervals along its length. The patient must place one finger in each successive space as he speaks—one word per 'space'.

3. A metronome may also be used to help the patient control his rate of utterance:

(i) He may be asked to speak each syllable (or single syllable word) to the beat of the metronome

(ii) As the patient improves, it may be possible to synchronize the *stressed syllables only,* with the beat of the metronome.

eg. a c̄up of t̄ea

ōpen the w̄indow

anōther p̄iece of c̄ake

h̄oover the c̄arpet

t̄wo ḡallons of p̄etrol

t̄here's s̄nooker on the t̄elevision.

4. Rhythmic cueing is recommended by Yorkston and Beukelman as a transition between the imposed control and the self-monitoring of rate. This is similar to the stress timing described in 3 (ii) above. However, in this instance the therapist indicates the pace at which the words should be read. This is done by pointing to the words instead of using the metronome. Patients are asked to follow the rhythm and the speed. The therapist may do one of the following:

(i) give the model for the patient to repeat

(ii) shadow-read with the patient, to reinforce the rhythm and control of the rate.

5. Berry and Goshorn (1981, 1983) describe the use of an oscilloscope display to give feedback to the patient. The patient is asked 'to 'fill-up' the five second window of oscilloscope display or to match slow productions of a target sentence'. He is encouraged to modify either pause time or articulation time so that he learns to control the rate of his utterance, making it last for the full five seconds of the visual oscilloscope display, thus matching the therapists's model.

This technique provides the patient with immediate feedback of rate control, and helps improve intelligibility.

6. Yorkston and Beukelman (1981) further suggest that it is important to establish 'optimum rate and intelligibility relationships'. By this they mean that patients are asked to 'reduce their speaking rate to the point at which their speech is 95% intelligible to the clinician'. A series of tape-recordings are made of the patient reading aloud. He is encouraged to alter his rate until the therapist can transcribe his speech from the recordings with 95% accuracy.

7. Another useful home practice exercise for patients working on rate is the development of 'sentence generation grids' (Yorkston and Beukelman, 1981). The patient is asked to create and practise reading aloud nonsense sentences from a grid. The grid contains the frame sentences: determiner+adjective+subject+verb+by the+object. Sentences are created by random selection of one word per column. Each column contains up to 50 words.

eg.

A	few	oranges	were thrown	by the boys
(determiner)	(col. 1)	(col. 2)	(col. 3)	(col. 4)

The patient then records these sentences and the next day listens to his own tape-recording and transcribes them. A small selection of words are given on page 79.

Exercises

Word list

(i)   /p/   /b/

       paint   bus
       paper   beach
       palace   brooch
       present   bruise
       prepare   black
       pleasant   blizzard

       /t/   /d/

       tongue   day
       tourist   deny
       tennis   describe
       towards   deliver
       try   dry
       treasure   drink

       /k/   /g/

       car   girl
       kennel   garage
       chemist   gossip
       curtain   grocer
       cry   grammar
       clear   glasses

       /m/   /n/

       many   no
       month   nation
       mimic   navy
       murmur   ninety
       minute   nonsense
       mischief   nuisance

/ŋ/

sing
fling
think
twinkle
sinking
beginning

/l/

lamb
lane
level
lonely
lovely
liberty

/r/

red
rain
rescue
referee
regret
register

/w/

week
wear
water
winter
wellington
weather

/f/

four
famous
forget
friction
frequent
flower

/v/

vent
vote
vehicle
valuable
vigorous
verify

/θ/	/ð/
thumb	that
thought	this
thunder	then
thirsty	therefore
thankyou	though
theatre	themselves

/s/	/z/
sand	zip
salt	zone
secret	zebra
science	zero
sausage	zodiac
search	xylophone

/ʃ/	/ʒ/
shell	pleasure
shoes	leisure
shop	casual
shoulder	treasure
shrub	erosion
shrink	visual

/tʃ/	/dʒ/
check	jam
cherry	juice
change	judge
chimney	journey
chinese	jealous
chestnut	journalist

(ii)   Random words for further practice for intelligibility.

pain	crunch	train
rock	crop	blare
square	swarm	rush
much	care	screw
stop	sneeze	lunch
push	still	sock
smoke	punch	cane
string	school	sleep
pear	prop	scratch
slight	scream	float
talk	bush	back
such	tear	scarlet
drop	touch	ground
snow	smart	mustard
lane	stitch	trouble
straight	rain	where
knock	spot	sand
swallow	track	limp
journal	choose	please
desk	glue	bloom

4-Word Sentences

Two pints of milk.
Come to the club.
Buy me a paper.
Put on the kettle.
A packet of cigarettes.
Go to the office.
Look at the *Radio Times*.
Switch on the television.
I'll take another photograph.
The dinner's getting burnt.

5-Word Sentences

He just didn't look well.
Try to work things out.
They'll never fit me now.
It was a great meeting.
She was not seriously injured.
I think I'm getting better.
I'm a very independent person.
My husband drives too fast.
We cooked carrots and onions.
He's earning a good salary.

6-Word Sentences

John took me out one day.
He asked me for a loan.
We all sat down and relaxed.
The programme is on later tonight.
I said I'd put on weight.
They have a lot of visitors.
How many hours have you worked?
They will spend the winter abroad.
The wallpaper is green and blue.
Four people worked in the restaurant.

7-Word Sentences

They had a good win on Saturday.
That's what life is really all about.
I saw him a few weeks later.
She suggested we all have dinner together.
Several paintings were sold at the auction.
Beans must be soaked and then cooked.
The office coffee machine was bubbling away.
We have to get the manager's permission.
Friday's a good night for watching television.
So why should anyone complain about that?

8-Word Sentences

I was pleased with the way things went.
I didn't know where they were coming from.
Travel is about the only leisure we have.
It was a huge part of my life.
The strike spread throughout much of the country.
Night after night they received anonymous phone calls.
He has only played football twice for England.
She washes her hair more often than necessary.
There's no admission charge but donations are accepted.
Enjoy the fine weather before the rain starts.

9-Word Sentences

I've been through too much to give in now.
You have a clear view almost all year long.
Eventually, of course, we all got used to it.
You must try to do whatever you think best.
For further details go on to the next page.
He said that he was too old to travel.
The police said the crash was not his fault.
The Prime Minister promised tax relief in the budget.
Every tourist wants to visit the Houses of Parliament.
The journey from England to Australia keeps getting shorter.

10-Word Sentences

These are some of the best vegetables and fruit available.
I looked for a flatmate to help with the bills.
Spending time with my family is really my favourite activity.
Fresh snow has fallen and the ski slopes are open.
Almost any day of the year is good for hiking.
Why would such a man be fired from his job?
That television programme is on every day of the week.
Nobody seemed to think he had such a terrible problem.
Few people could say no to such a kind invitation.
The noise from the exhaust pipe grew louder and louder.

‘DON’T ENCOURAGE DRINKERS’ – WARNING

Publicans have been told not to encourage young drinkers who face the dangers of becoming chronic alcoholics in later life, if they drink to excess now.

And licensees have been told they will lose their licence if found guilty of serving under-age drinkers or serving after hours.

Sheila Humphreys, chairman of the licensing justices, told last week’s annual general licensing meeting at Knutsford that licensees must be aware of under-age drinkers – particularly licensees who run off-licences.

‘We know that pressure upon licensees is very great, particularly with under-age and after hours drinking,’ she said. ‘Licensees have a big responsibility in the community. A majority of crimes are committed whilst under the influence of alcohol and often by the under-18’s.’

Mrs Humphreys went on to warn against the dangers of excessive drinking.

‘Youthful drinking can lead to chronic alcoholism in later life and we would urge licensees to particularly keep their eye on young drinkers – and older drinkers – and not to serve them to excess.’

2 SWEET DREAMS OF THE PAST

Too much strain on the heart is not a good thing, but a little heart-fluttering on St Valentine's Day never did anybody any harm. It is pleasant to receive a romantic card, a posy of flowers or to cook a special meal for the one you love.

But in the last century, St Valentine's Eve was also important to maidens and bachelors because it was a time to look into the future.

The object was to discover who you were going to marry and also whether the nuptials would occur during the year. One method, said to be infallible, was to hard-boil an egg, remove the yolk, fill the cavity with salt and then eat the white, the salt and the shell, without either speaking or drinking afterwards. If you dreamt of your sweetheart, then all would be well. There is no record of what to expect if you had a nightmare!

You could, if you preferred, take five bay leaves, pin one to each corner of your pillow and the fifth in the middle, then lie down and sleep. This way, should you dream of your loved one, you would know you would be wed before Christmas.

3 CHEF'S CHOICE

Sweet Pancakes (for four people)

Pancake Mix

4 oz plain flour
1 egg
½ oz butter
½ pint of milk
2 oz lard
Pinch of salt
Tablespoon of sugar

1. Whisk the egg, salt, milk and sugar together, add sieved flour a little at a time.

2. Whisk in the melted butter and pour the mixture through the strainer and leave to stand.
   It is worth noting that the batter will benefit from standing for a couple of hours.

Cooking method

1. Melt lard in a heated pan, pour off the excess, pour mixture into pan to a thickness of ¼″. Cook until golden brown, making sure pan does not become over-heated.

2. Flip pancake over and repeat the process.

And now for the filling:

Crepe Suzette

¼ oz butter
¼ oz sugar
1 lemon
1 orange
1 measure Grand Marnier

Method

1. Grate orange and lemon and retain the zest and juice.

2. Melt butter and sugar in a pan, add juice and zest and bring to the boil.

3. Add the folded pancakes and pour in Grand Marnier and flame.

4 STARTING FROM SCRATCH

There is always great excitement when moving into a new house. I remember well when we moved into ours here in Shropshire in 1963. There is an enormous amount to think of, and so much to be done.

Quite naturally when you move house or buy your first home, there are the contents and fittings to be given first priority, and there is so much expense in the early stages. The garden must take second place. But how sickening to look out on bare earth, or possibly builders' rubble and all that goes with it.

Far too often with gardens of new houses there is a mere covering of soil over the rubble or the hard-packed ground where bulldozers and other machinery have been trundling about. It is a heart-breaking task to have to face.

The garden can only be done in stages, and this is the way I would prefer to do it anyway.

Let's first of all consider the tools and equipment. The essentials are a spade, fork, rake and hoe, and most gardening operations can be done with these basic tools.

My advice is always to buy good garden tools: cheap tools are not a good investment. If good garden tools are looked after, kept clean and occasionally wiped over with an oily rag and stored in the dry, they will last almost a lifetime. Once you have the basics, your garden tools ought to extend to a trowel, a pair of secateurs, garden shears and a lawn mower. There are so many gadgets on the market to avoid in the early stages. These can come later, if and when they may be required.

Starting with a raw new house garden, my first requirement would be to have the whole area made clean and tidy. Any bricks, mortar, stones and other rubble I would clear to one corner. There is no point in having them taken away; they could come in useful for making garden paths, etc. My advice is to have the area cleared and cultivated and sown down with grass seed, which would not be too expensive. It may be necessary to get a contractor with a rotary cultivator, as breaking up impacted soil can be very hard work. Follow that advice and all that will be necessary is to keep the grass mown, and you will be looking out on a tidy, restful area.

5 TAILOR-MADE HOLIDAYS

When you book with Eurocamp, your holiday package is put together especially for you. We don't try to fit people into a set formula because we know everyone wants something different.

Our flexible system means that you can set off on any day of the week, have any length of holiday, with prices adjusted accordingly. And there's a complete range of cross-channel ferry services to choose from. You just select your date, time and point of departure and we do the rest.

You can stop off at a hotel or one of our overnight camp sites. Or if you prefer, we can arrange Motorail for your journey. Just tell us what you want then sit back and let us do the work. It's a completely tailor-made holiday.

6 A HOLIDAY IN FRANCE

A great spider's web of rivers wind their way across the ancient province of Aquitane which covers much of south-west France. The Charente and Dordogne rivers meander through lovely undulating countryside – a countryside with so much history and so much that is typical of the real France.

Few of France's many rivers are better known or better loved than the Dordogne. Where else but here, in this beautiful countryside, along the river's sun-dappled banks, would you ever find the prehistoric caves, medieval castles, pretty stone villages, the river beaches for swimming and canoeing, the superb country restaurants, and the quite exceptional campsites, that together make the Dordogne unique?

When all is said and done, though, the enduring memory is of the rivers themselves, enchanting all who follow their meandering way through villages splashed with flowers, beneath the gaze of proud cliff-top castles. From the shade of cafe terraces the view falls on a manor house half hidden in the trees; a fisherman perhaps; the eddy of a canoe that passes. Along the river banks are meadows for a midday picnic and beaches from which to swim. In the evening there are restaurants, tucked away in country villages, serving the specialities which make the region a paradise for lovers of good food.

7 ESCORT CABRIOLET

Ford's classy Cabriolet combines the fun of open-air motoring with room for all the family.

The new Escort Cabriolet is a brilliant blend of open-topped sporting car and practical, family-sized saloon. It combines all the fun-in-the-sun characteristics of a roof-down roadster with seats for up to five people, plenty of luggage space, and a snug-fitting roof that's notably quick and easy to operate.

Although based on the award-winning Escort – Britain's most popular car – the eye-catching Cabriolet has many unique features. Designing an open model involves a great deal more than just removing the steel roof and replacing it with a fabric hood. That's why Ford spent more than three years perfecting a car that's every bit as strong as its saloon and estate counterparts in the front-wheel-drive Escort range.

8 TODAY'S CARS

There are many cars in the Ford model range.

They extend from the small but roomy Fiesta to the elegant, luxurious Granada.

Each of the six families in the Ford range – Fiesta, Escort, Capri, Orion, Sierra and Granada – is painstakingly planned and backed by Britain's best service network.

Each has an outstanding selection of trim, equipment, engines and transmissions, so that individual needs can be matched. Beyond the standard engines, each family is available with specially-developed powertrains – offering remarkable economy or scintillating performance. For instance, the Fiesta 1.1 with an optional five-speed manual gearbox returns an official 58.9 mpg at a steady 56 mph while the Capri 2.8 Injection's power-packed V6 takes it effortlessly to 130 mph. In the Sierra and Granada, diesel engines supplement the wide range of petrol engines.

Sentence Frame

A/The + (Adjective) + (Subject) + were + (Verb) + by the + (Object)

big	orange(s)	thrown	boys
silver	pea(s)	tossed	men
few	walnut(s)	cooked	neighbour
real	table(s)	sold	secretary
free	ball(s)	packed	ladies
hidden	cake(s)	taken	farmer
small	telephone(s)	left	family
black	pencil(s)	lost	policeman
round	box(es)	read	girls
sweet	book(s)	given	friend
green	pepper(s)	eaten	chef
plastic	coin(s)	removed	butcher

CHAPTER 11
PROSODY

'Prosody may be defined as the patterned distribution of stress, intonation and other phonatory features in speech. In effective oral communication, the prosodic and suprasegmental features of intonation, tone of the voice and stress contribute greatly to the determination of the implied meaning and to the overall intelligibility of the speaker.'

(Scott, Caird and Williams, 1985)

'From the phonetic point of view, prosodic features may be defined as vocal effects constituted by variations along the parameters of pitch, loudness, duration and silence.'

(Crystal, 1969)

From these definitions, it is apparent that the suprasegmentals of English cover a whole range of vocal parameters, and that their appropriate and accurate usage are vital to the overall effectiveness of the speaker's communication.

Prosody, therefore, is not 'the icing on the cake' which it was once considered. It does in fact 'make a significant contribution to the intelligibility of speech'. (Darwin, 1975).

Disturbance of prosody is present in all dysarthric speech and, in fact, is particularly diagnostic in the case of ataxic and hypokinetic dysarthrias, of which it is a prominent feature. Because normal prosody requires precise co-ordination of all the speech processes, ataxic dysarthric speakers have particular problems, since their neurological deficits are related to a lack of co-ordination of neuro-muscular activity. One of the net results of the Parkinson's disease patient's festinant pattern of movement is a tendency towards palilalia and hence disintegrated prosody.

Rosenbek and La Pointe (1978) state that English has three prosodic features: rhythm, stress and intonation. This chapter seeks to provide some systematic therapy to facilitate the correct use of these prosodic features.

Rhythm and Stress

Rhythm is the timing of speech resulting in part from changes in pause time.

Stress is also related in part to changes in pause time, but it also implies changes in pitch, loudness and articulation time.

It is difficult to separate rhythm and stress because they are so dependent on each other. Therapy, therefore, treats both with a common method. The value of working on rhythm and stress is commented on by Yorkston and Beukelman (1981):

'Forcing marginally intelligible speakers into specific stress patterns tends to increase intelligibility and reduce bizarreness.'

1. *Respiratory control*—'Control and modification of the expiratory phase of respiration produces the stress contrasts in speech and the regular temporal patterns of stressed and unstressed syllables that result in the characteristic rhythm of English.' (Grunwell and Huskins, 1979).

It is therefore important to practise the breathing exercises outlined in Chapter 6 not only to support phonation and articulation, but also to provide the basis for rhythm and stress control.

2. To facilitate *rhythmic control* ask the patient to read rhymes, poems and limericks that have a very strong beat. (A metronome, clapping or a pen tapping will provide the basic beat.)

The cautionary verses of Hilaire Belloc and Edward Lear's nonsense rhymes, have proved suitable material and also introduce an element of fun and humour into the therapy session. Two examples will be found on page 82.

3. Luria (1970), in discussion of intersystemic reorganization, encourages the pairing of speaking with another activity, such as button pushing, ball squeezing or tapping. Any of these may be used in conjunction with the above exercises or with most of the following rhythm and stress work.

Scott and Caird (1981) have described the benefits of using the Vocalite (a voice operated light source) which responds to changes in stress and acts as a visual monitor and reinforcer of prosodic aspects of the patient's own speech.

4. Contrastive stress drill, after Fairbanks, described in detail by Rosenbek and La Pointe (1978), has been shown by many clinicians to encourage more appropriate stress patterns in speech. 'The nucleus of the drill is composed of two or more stimuli that are different in meaning because of differences in stress. For example, the meaning of 'Bill bit Bob' depends on whether primary stress falls on the first, second or third word. See exercises on page 83.

5. To carry over contrastive stress drills into conversational speech, the clinician should embark on a style of dialogue similar to those outlined in the previous section. This time, *the patient will answer the questions in his own words.* Two examples are given below.

Where were you **born?**	I was **born** in **London.**
Were you born in **Manchester**?	No, I was born in **London**.
Was your **wife** born in London?	No, I was born in London.
Do you **live** in London?	No, I was **born** in London.
What **sport** do you like?	I like **football**.
Do you like **golf**?	No, I like **football**.
Does your **wife** like football?	No, **I** like football.

Although the patient may not answer with the exact words suggested above, the therapist's questions should be framed to facilitate responses that require a variety of marked stress patterns. There should be a pause prior to each of the patient's responses to allow him time to think up his answer and rehearse it silently before saying it aloud.

6. When the concepts of rhythm and stress have been established, then exercises can be given that involve the patient in recognizing and monitoring stress patterns in normal, everyday conversational speech and reading.

The patient and therapist together should mark the stressed words in everyday phrases and sentences; and in prose extracts. Then the patient reads aloud the sentences and the prose passages with the correct stress. Some examples of sentences and prose passages are given on page 84.

The passages on page 85 have been marked for stress to assist the patient in identifying the naturally stressed syllables and words.

Intonation

Netsell (1973) defines intonation as 'the perception of changes in the fundamental frequency of vocal fold vibration'. This places intonation firmly within the realms of phonation; some exercises for improving intonation have been described in Chapter 7.

However, it is appropriate that intonation practice should also be described in a chapter on prosody. Intonation not only implies a neurophysiological change in vocal fold vibration but it is also a linguistically based parameter (Grunwell and Huskins, 1979). It alters according to the mood and feeling the speaker wants to convey.

The normal terminal intonation pattern in a simple declarative and imperative sentence in English is falling, eg. I am going home. ↓ On the other hand, questions that can be answered by 'yes' or 'no' have a terminal intonation that rises, eg. Am I right? ↑

As good respiratory control is a prerequisite for rhythm and stress, so good phonatory control is necessary for efficient intonational change.

Intonation exercises

1. Ask the patient to practise the rising and falling intonation patterns on a simple vowel sound (as described in Chapter 7).

eg. /a: .../ ↗

/a: .../ ↘

/a: .../ ↗↘

/a: .../ ↘↗

2. Illustrate to the patient how different emotions can be conveyed through differing intonation patterns.

Give the patient a model and then ask him to try to imitate the different intonation patterns and hence convey the emotion.

eg.   (i) excited
  (ii) bored
  (iii) happy
  (iv) sad
  (v) angry
  (vi) frustrated
  (vii) puzzled
  (viii) bitter
  (ix) disappointed
  (x) encouraging

These emotions may be conveyed using a single exclamatory 'Oh' with the varying intonational changes or they may be conveyed using a whole meaningful utterance.

eg.   (i) I am so excited about my holiday next week.
  (ii) I am fed up doing this every day.
  (iii) I love every aspect of my life.
  (iv) I was sorry to hear about your mother.
  (v) I am furious that they have sent that bill again.
  (vi) I just cannot seem to make him understand.
  (vii) I don't know what you mean.
  (viii) I will never understand why he did that.
  (ix) I can't believe he would let us down.
  (x) Let's try it all over again.

3. Practise terminal intonation on a series of simple, declarative and imperative sentences. (These all require falling intonation on the final word in the sentence.)

eg. I think you are right. ↓
The man walked his dog round the park. ↓
The children are playing in the garden. ↓
Go and sit down! ↓
Don't say another word! ↓
Give me that book! ↓

4. Practise terminal intonation on a series of 'yes' or 'no' questions. (These all require rising intonation on the final word of the question.)

eg. Do you like fish? ↑
May I come in? ↑
Is this your car? ↑
Do you come here often? ↑
Is that your wife over there? ↑

Exercises

'JIM' BY HILAIRE BELLOC

There was a Boy whose name was Jim;
His Friends were very good to him.
They gave him Tea, and Cakes, and Jam,
And slices of delicious Ham,
And Chocolate with pink inside,
And little Tricycles to ride,
And read him stories through and through,
And even took him to the Zoo –
But there it was the dreadful Fate
Befell him, which I now relate.

You know at least you ought to know,
For I have often told you so –
That children never are allowed
To leave their Nurses in a Crowd;
Now this was Jim's especial Foible,
He ran away when he was able,
And on this inauspicious day
He slipped his hand and ran away!

LIMERICKS BY EDWARD LEAR

There was an old man with a beard,
Who said, 'It is just as I feared! –
Two owls and a Hen,
Four Larks and a Wren,
Have all built their nests in my beard!'

There was a young lady from Ryde,
Whose shoestrings were seldom untied;
She purchased some clogs
And some spotty dogs,
And frequently walked about Ryde.

This drill is usually conducted as a dialogue. The words to be stressed are **printed in bold type.**

	Therapist	**Patient**
1.	Bill bit Bob.	Bill bit Bob.
	Who bit Bob?	**Bill** bit Bob.
	Did **Bob** bite Bill?	No, **Bill** bit Bob.
	Did Bill bite **Tom**?	No, Bill bit **Bob**.
2.	The dog chased the cat.	The dog chased the cat.
	Who chased the cat?	The **dog** chased the cat.
	Did the **cat** chase the **dog**?	No, the **dog** chased the **cat**.
	Did the dog chase the **mouse**?	No, the dog chased the **cat**.
3.	Jim scored three goals.	Jim scored three goals.
	Who scored three goals?	**Jim** scored three goals.
	Did Jim score **two** goals?	No, Jim scored **three** goals.
	Did Jim **save** three goals?	No, Jim **scored** three goals.
	Did **Paul** score three goals?	No, **Jim** scored three goals.
4.	Jill made a pot of tea.	Jill made a pot of tea.
	Who made a pot of tea?	**Jill** made a pot of tea.
	Did Jill make a pot of **coffee**?	No, Jill made a pot of **tea**.
	Did Jill make a **cup** of tea?	No, Jill made a **pot** of tea.
	Did **Mary** make a pot of tea?	No, **Jill** made a pot of tea.
5.	Dick bought two gallons of petrol.	Dick bought two gallons of petrol.
	Who bought two gallons of petrol?	**Dick** bought two gallons of petrol.
	Did Dick **steal** two gallons of petrol?	No, Dick **bought** two gallons of petrol.
	Did Dick buy **four** gallons of petrol?	No, Dick bought **two** gallons of petrol.
	Did Dick buy two gallons of **oil**?	No, Dick bought two gallons of **petrol**.

(a) He's playing **foot**ball on **Sat**urday.

John drove **all** the **way** to **Ab**erdeen.

They are **com**ing to fit the **car**pet on **Tues**day.

Let's have a cup of **coffee** before going **home**.

The **weather man** said it would **rain** today.

(b) Ambiguous sentences can be used where a change of stress can change the meaning or mood of the whole sentence, eg:

I want you to come with me:

I want you to come with me.

I **want** you to come with me.

I want you to come **with** me.

I want you to come with **me**.

John is coming to tea on Sunday:

John is coming to tea on Sunday.

John **is** coming to tea on Sunday.

John is coming to **tea** on Sunday.

John is coming to tea on **Sunday**.

INSIDE A VOLCANO

When it `first broke away from the `sun, the `earth was a
`great `ball of `fire, `mostly made up of `burning `gases. As it
`cooled, the `outside `hardened into `rock, but the `inside is
`still `red `hot. `Deep beneath the `surface of the `earth lie
`great `quantities of `molten `rock. This is under `great
`pressure and is `usually `trapped by the `earth's `crust.
When a `crack appears in the `crust, perhaps as the re`sult of
an `earthquake, the `molten `rock in the form of `lava, `forces
its `way `through to `form a vol`cano.

Al`though e`rupting vol`canoes do a `great `deal of `damage,
we can `learn a `lot about the `centre of the `earth by
`studying them and the `lava and `gases they throw `out.

FRUITS AND SEEDS

When `eating `sweet and `juicy `strawberries, have you ever
`stopped and `wondered why the `plant has made such a
`tasty and `tempting `fruit?

`This `plant has `one main `job each `summer, to `try to
`spread its `seeds as `far away as `possible. What a `problem
this is, because the `plant can `hardly `move at `all! In`stead
it produces a `brightly `coloured `fruit with `seeds on the
`outside. `Usually it is `not `long before the `fruit is `seen and
`taken away. Just a `few of those `tiny `seeds will find a `new
`place to `grow, `sometimes `many `miles from the `parent
`plant.

`Many plants rely on `humans, `animals or `birds to disperse
their `seeds, but the `poppy uses the `wind. When the `plant
`sways in the `wind, `tiny `seeds are sent `spilling from the
`poppy-`head. The `seeds may travel only a `few `inches, but
this is `far enough for `some to `reach a `place where they can
`grow.

CHAPTER 12
SUMMARY

Our concept of the nature of dysarthria has grown and developed in recent years. We now identify different types of dysarthria (viz. flaccid, spastic, ataxic, hypokinetic, hyperkinetic and mixed) that can cause widespread disruptions of a whole range of parameters (viz. respiration, phonation, articulation, prosody etc.). And we have also become increasingly aware of the more holistic approach required in therapy.

The preceding chapters of this book have described in detail a range of exercises specifically designed to rehabilitate the defective motor speech parameters. In our consideration of whole patient management there are, however, a number of additional factors that should be considered and incorporated into therapy.

Motivation and Mood

Most writers on the topic of dysarthria refer at some point to the need for high motivation in therapy. If this motivation can emanate from patient, relatives and therapists alike, then the optimum environment is assured. However, all those working with dysarthrics recognise that a lack of motivation is intrinsic to some neurological conditions. In addition to what may be described as 'normal' depression resulting from a progressive or chronic disability, therapists will have observed the specific lack of drive which may occur in Parkinson's Disease; the occurrence of depression after the sudden onset of a stroke and its debilitating effects; and the emotional lability which is so characteristic of the patient with Pseudo-bulbar palsy.

It is important, therefore, that the therapist sees herself in the role of encourager and motivator, endeavouring to lead the patient through the minefield of depression, tearfulness and dejection. While a positive and cheerful approach to therapy cannot guarantee success, and the presence of depression should not be ignored but acknowledged, constructive rehabilitation can best be achieved in an optimistic atmosphere.

Groups

Perhaps the most stimulating and motivating setting for dysarthria therapy is a dysarthria group. The authors, in Chapter 13, report on the positive effects for Parkinson's Disease patients, of being treated in groups of 5 to 8. The cumulative effect of each individual's drive and motivation and the general desire to communicate and to be understood, add to the effectiveness of such therapy sessions.

The routine drills of respiration, phonation or prosody exercises, for example, lend themselves to group participation and response. In addition, patients gain insight into their own and others' problems while the potential tedium of learning and practising techniques of breathing, for example, is relieved.

In addition the group setting presents a perfect opportunity for techniques, rehearsed within the 'vacuum' of an exercise, to be put to immediate functional use. The presence of the therapist and other members of the group ensures positive feedback on progress. It also provides the listening dysarthrics with valuable practice in analysis and constructive criticism.

A wide range of group activities may be organised which will provide interest, incentive and invaluable practice.

These may include: play reading
interviewing
engaging in dialogue
role play
chairing quizzes
calling 'Bingo'
delivering instructive talks
going out on 'assignments'

Environmental Education

Thus far we have concentrated our attention on treating the dysarthric patient; but Berry and Sanders, in their contribution to Berry's *Clinical Dysarthria* (1983), emphasize the concept of Environmental Education. This concept means that not only the patient but also those around him are made aware of factors within the environment that can help or hinder his communication and, in particular, his intelligibility.

Noise, for example, in the immediate vicinity of the dysarthric speaker will interfere with intelligibility. Advise the patient, if the noise is variable, to turn it down; if the noise cannot be controlled, move away from its source and move closer to the listener, rather than try to speak louder; and ensure that the listener is watching.

Lighting, too, is an important consideration, so teach the patient to sit in a well-lit area so that the listener can see his face. Ensure that, in a group conversation, all the listeners have a full-face view of the speaker.

Resonance factors must also be understood. Noise dampening by carpets and heavy curtains will allow the patient to speak at a lower volume, whereas in a large bare room with hard walls the acoustic will be very different. In the latter setting, the dysarthric speaker should move closer to his listener who will need to attend more closely to visual cues such as gesture and facial expression.

Where it is possible and profitable, the patient should be encouraged to use external aids to facilitate intelligibility. A voice amplifier may be supplied to a dysarthric if his speech is characterized by reduced volume; and if the patient's spouse is hard of hearing, he or she should be encouraged to wear a hearing aid.

Telephone amplifiers are also available to boost either the signal of the sender or of the receiver.

Berry and Sanders further indicate the advisability of completing a 'situational intelligibility survey' which analyses the situations where a patient's speech is found least intelligible (eg. when watching television; in the car; in a restaurant). They also list 'suggestions to improve your communication', which they recommend giving to patients. These give hints on how to cope in noisy situations, on the telephone etc.

In conclusion, management of the dysarthric patient involves more than symptomatic treatment of motor speech parameters. It also implies the manipulation of the patient's environment, the counselling of relatives and friends within his close social circle, and the integration of therapy into all communication situations.

CHAPTER 13
EFFICACY OF SPEECH THERAPY

This chapter aims to draw the reader's attention to recent evidence of successful therapy with some groups of dysarthrics. It is hoped that more therapists will feel encouraged to tackle the onorous task of treating patients with dysarthria, including those suffering from progressive neurological conditions.

It must be acknowledged that there is a paucity of such studies documented in the literature, but the few referred to below serve to lay the foundations of a positive approach to the challenge of treating dysarthric patients. The studies themselves will also indicate the value of different therapeutic techniques and may lead therapists to experiment with their own approach to management and therapy.

The efficacy and long-term effects of intensive treatment in Parkinson's Disease

The authors' own recent research findings in the field of Parkinson's Disease highlight the positive immediate results and long-term benefits of intensive speech therapy. This study is reported in detail in the British Journal of Disorders of Communication (Vol. 19, 213–224, 1984).

A total of 18 patients with Parkinson's Disease were able to complete all the necessary stages of assessment and hence provide the data for the results. Twelve of the patients were randomly allocated to two treatment groups and participated in a two-week intensive speech therapy programme. The other six formed a control group.

The treatment groups were assessed on three occasions: immediately prior to therapy; immediately following a two-week period of intensive therapy; and after a period of three months without further therapy. The control group were assessed at the same intervals, but did not receive any therapy during the period of the study.

The treatment group each received approximately 35 to 40 hours of therapy during the two-week period (an average of 3½ to 4 hours per day as an out-patient in a hospital setting). The programme consisted of group sessions at the beginning of each morning to improve method, capacity and control of breathing; co-ordination and control of voice production (with particular emphasis on pitch variation and loudness); range, strength and speed of articulatory muscle movement; articulation; control of rate of speech; variation of intonation and stress patterns; and overall intelligibility of communication.

This was followed by individual sessions for some patients as required and by further group sessions designed to encourage patients to listen carefully and monitor each other's performance, through play reading, video recording, etc. The afternoon sessions were much less structured and formal, with activities ranging from discussions, quizzes and speech making, to interviewing and role play. These were intended to facilitate the functional application of therapeutic techniques.

The results of this study suggest that speech therapy, given on an intensive daily basis for a period of 2 weeks, is of benefit to Parkinson's Disease patients. A previous study undertaken by the authors (Robertson and Thomson, 1983) had indicated the benefits of intensive residential therapy. This more recent study underlined the benefits of intensive therapy in a non-residential, hospital-based setting.

Improvement was evident in almost every aspect of motor speech production and related activities. These included respiration, phonation, movement of the facial musculature, reflex activity for coughing and swallowing, articulation, intelligibility, and the prosodic aspects of stress, intonation and rate.

The results further indicated that the patients not only showed measurable improvement immediately following a period of therapy, but also that they were able to maintain this improvement. In some cases, it was apparent that improvement continued even after a period of three months without therapy.

The implication for the practising speech therapist may be that, while neither discharge nor weekly therapy are appropriate to the needs of such patients (Allen, 1970), it may be of great benefit to set up two-week intensive therapy programmes for a group of patients two or three times a year. This, it is suggested, could increase the patients' motivation, encourage them to maintain their communicative abilities and ensure that the patients have accurate knowledge of techniques they could practise at home. They would also have expert professional monitoring of their speech on a fairly regular basis.

The effects of Prosodic Therapy for Parkinson's Disease Patients

Scott and Caird have reported in several recent publications on the efficacy of a therapy programme for Parkinson's Disease patients. Treatment given concentrated almost exclusively on the prosodic aspects of the patients' dysarthria (see British Medical Journal, 24 Oct. 1981, 283, 1088 and Communication in Parkinson's Disease, Scott, Caird & Williams, 1985).

Twenty-six P.D. patients with speech disorders received daily prosodic exercise therapy at home for two or three weeks. The main focus of therapy was on intonation, stress and rhythm, and was aimed at increasing the patient's awareness of the abnormal prosodic features of his own speech. Practice in more normal patterns of conversational speech was encouraged. This was supplemented by a voice-operated visual reinforcement device, the Vocalite.

The results indicated a significant improvement in speech production and, in addition, increased awareness of the prosodic features in the speech of others. This improvement was maintained, in part, for up to three months. Small changes in prosodic abnormality could, in individual patients, be associated with substantial improvement in social communication. The use of the visual reinforcement device produced limited benefit over and above that of exercise alone, except among those patients with severe speech disorders.

This study has several implications for the practising speech therapist. Firstly, it emphasizes the benefits of domiciliary therapy, as all the patients were treated in their own homes. Secondly, treatment, though regarded as 'intensive', amounted to only one hour per day, which is much less than the amount discussed in the previous study.

Ataxic Dysarthria: Treatment Sequences Based on Intelligibility and Prosodic Considerations

Much of the recent work of Yorkston and Beukelman has concentrated on the assessment and treatment of intelligibility in dysarthric patients. This study, reported in detail in the Journal of Speech and Hearing Disorders (Vol. 46, 398–404, Nov. 1981), was concerned with designing and assessing the efficacy of a treatment programme for four ataxic dysarthric speakers.

The four subjects described in the paper exhibited sudden, adult onset of ataxic dysarthria. None of the subjects had degenerative cerebellar disease. Speech treatment was initiated two to six weeks post-onset and continued until eight to ten months post-onset. Initially, the speech intelligibility scores of all subjects were less than 30% and speaking rates were in excess of 100 words per minute for oral reading tasks. Prosodic patterns were also markedly abnormal, illustrating the susceptibility of ataxic dysarthric patients to problems and deficits in this area.

A hierarchy of rate control strategies, ranging from rigid imposition of rate, through rhythmic cueing to self-monitored rate control, formed the basis for therapy. Treatment, primarily designed to improve prosody, was initiated after speech intelligibility had reached the target level consistently.

The individual progress of each of the patients is given in some detail in the paper. Individual goals were set and achieved, with modification of techniques made to suit individual needs.

The treatment approach of this study was necessitated by the unique pattern of ataxic speakers, whose chief deficit appears to be co-ordination of speech process components rather than deficits specific to certain points along the vocal tract. This overall approach must, of course, be supplemented by attention to particular features where specific problem areas can be identified.

The results of the study do justify the use of rate control strategies to aid intelligibility. This is an area which the authors believe has hitherto received insufficient attention.

CHAPTER 14
AIDS TO COMMUNICATION

The field of communication aids and alternative systems is one which is expanding at an ever-increasing rate as our knowledge of the nature of speech disorders improves, and as the relevant technologies continue to advance. Reference has been made in previous chapters to a number of electronic and mechanical devices which may be regarded as general aids to communication or as specific therapeutic aids or adjuncts to therapy.

It is not possible to do justice to this subject in the space available. Therefore, readers are urged to refer to the texts recommended at the end of this book, and to consult their nearest Communication Aids Centre both for specific assessment and for more general advice. A list of these is given at the end of this chapter.

There is potential for the use of a variety of signing systems, charts and gadgets when treating dysarthric patients. The choice will depend upon a multiplicity of factors, including the exact nature and severity of the patient's speech problem, his specific communication needs, the likely course of his disorder, and the demands of his environment. Palatal lift devices, voice amplifiers and electronic speech substitutes are among the range of options, while drool-control systems, the laryngo-scope and other monitors of vocal performance and nasality, may be employed as an integral part of a therapy programme.

In order to avoid any possible suspicion that the introduction of alternative means of communication may indicate a failure in the patients attempts to regain speech, it is advisable to introduce these early on, as part of the wider treatment plan. If a system or gadget is introduced too abruptly, and after a period of therapy without aids, it may be rejected. In this event, the relationship with the therapist could be adversely affected.

Schiefelbusch (1980) suggests several criteria for introducing a communication aid:

1. An alternative system can be used as part of the diagnostic procedure to determine patterns of functioning.

2. A system may provide the individual with the mechanism for expressing needs.

3. A system may provide a basis for the establishment of functional language process.

4. It may be used to supplement or strengthen oral language skills.

5. It may provide a means of expressive communication for an unintelligible patient.

An additional advantage to the use of an aid, is that the patient's oral skills tend to improve when the pressure for intelligible speech is reduced. This may be attributable to lessening of physical effort but also reflects the relief of frustration at not always being understood. For the dysarthric, in particular, these factors are very significant: increased effort and tension tend to impede satisfactory speech production.

I. Signs and Symbols

There are several sign and symbol systems in use in the United Kingdom. These include Amer-Ind, Bliss, Makaton, Paget Gorman Sign System and Rebus. Some of these are being used with patients with acquired dysarthria, although their primary use is with children who have developmental speech and language problems. Readers are referred to an article in the College of Speech Therapists' Bulletin (Thomson, May 1982). Further details of these systems can be obtained from your nearest Communication Aids Centre.

2. Charts

Communication charts are usually divided into sections, each containing a symbol, letter, word, picture, number or common phrase, depending on the needs and abilities of the user. There are commercially produced charts available (eg. from Winslow Press, the College of Speech Therapists, and the Chest, Heart and Stroke Association – for further information contact the Communication Aids Centres); however, many therapists prefer to make their own, so that the size and shape of the board and the vocabulary selection are suited to each individual patient.

3. Electronic Aids

These can be divided into groups according to their size, what they do and the way in which they are operated. They can be considered to be 'portable', 'less portable', or 'non-portable', and a description of aids under these headings is available in the RICA booklet *Communication Aids,* 1984.

Operation of electronic aids is often open to adaptation, but they are operated by pointing directly with the finger, or by use of a head-pointer, eye-pointing, or specific hand- or foot-operated switches. A range of switches is available and it is important to find the most consistent, reliable mode of access for each patient. Output may be in print or by visual display or voice synthesis; however, some aids combine more than one mode of output.

Assessment

Assessment is vital prior to the provision of any additional or alternative means of communication. When assessing the individual with dysarthria, reference should be made to the medical history and, in particular, to the onset and likely progression of the disorder. Current physical and intellectual abilities, speech and language levels, visual and hearing acuity and discrimination must be taken into account, along with the patient's overall communicative ability. The choice of an aid will also be influenced by his specific needs and the environment in which he lives and/or works.

It may also become clear, from the information gathered, that the individual will need more than one aid (eg. a non-portable aid at work and a portable aid at all other times). Where a patient's disorder is of a progressive nature, as in Motor Neurone Disease, the individual's abilities and needs must be continually reassessed, different aids being provided as and when necessary.

The therapist must consider whether the aid will be used as the primary means of communication or as a supplementary technique. Some individuals are able to communicate effectively with family and friends, but need an additional system for other environments. Aids may also be issued on a temporary basis while a dysarthric is working to improve oral skills.

Assessment of aids themselves should take account of factors such as the rate of transmission, error rate, intelligibility and/or visibility of the message, practicality and reliability as well as the initial cost and the maintenance service offered.

Training

When all other factors have been accounted for, an alternative or additional means of communication will only be effective if both the user and the people within the immediate environment are motivated to initiate and receive communication by this channel and are trained to use the system properly. It is essential for the patient to know how to operate the aid and how to cope with the practical details, such as charging the batteries or replacing the paper spool. Practice under supervision is important, too, so that competence and speed can be built up, and any problems that arise can be dealt with immediately. In this way, the aid is more likely to be used to the full. Without adequate training and support, a patient may abandon his aid because it is found 'too difficult'.

Provision

Communication aids can be provided by the NHS, but a consultant's prescription is required. The Communication Aids Centres in the United Kingdom (see below) are able to assess and recommend aids for patients, but do not have fundings to buy the aids. These Centres have a library loans service from which a recommended aid can be borrowed for a period of time. The CACs will only accept referral for assessment if provision for funding has already been established. Other sources of funding include Local Education

Authorities (for children of school age), Social Services Departments, and charities such as SEQUAL (formerly PUA), and CASH.

Communication Aids Centres

London:

(i) Communication Aids Centre,
Wolfson Centre,
Mecklenburgh Square,
LONDON WC1N 2AP.
(children)

(ii) Communication Aids Centre,
Charing Cross Hospital,
Fulham Palace Road,
LONDON W6 8RF.
(adults)

Bristol:

Communication Aids Centre,
Speech Therapy Department,
Frenchay Hospital,
BRISTOL BS16 1LE.
(adults mainly)

Cardiff:

Communication Aids Centre,
Rookwood Hospital,
Fairwater Road,
Llandaff,
CARDIFF CF5 2YN.
Wales
(adults and, predominantly, children)

Midlands:

Communication Aids Centre,
Boulton Road,
WEST BROMWICH,
West Midlands B70 6NN.
(adults and children)

Belfast:

Communication Aids Centre,
Prosthetic Orthotic and Aids Service,
Musgrave Park Hospital,
Stockman's Lane,
BELFAST B19 7JB.

Newcastle:

Communication Aids Centre,
Royal Victoria Infirmary,
Queen Victoria Road,
NEWCASTLE-UPON-TYNE NE2 4HH.
(adults and children)

BIBLIOGRAPHY

Allen, C M, 'Treatment of non-fluent speech resulting from neurological disease: Treatment of dysarthria'; *British Journal of Disorders of Communication,* 5, 3–5, 1970.

Berry, W R & Goshorn, E L, 'Immediate visual feedback in the treatment of ataxic dysarthria: a case study'; in *Clinical Dysarthria,* edited by W Berry, College-Hill Press, 1983.

Berry, W R & Goshorn, E L, *'Oscilloscopic feedback in the treatment of ataxic dysarthria',* cited in 'Ataxic Dysarthria: Treatment sequences based on intelligibility and prosodic considerations', *Journal of Speech and Hearing Disorders,* 46, 398–404, 1981.

Boone, D R, *The Voice and Voice Therapy,* 3rd edition, Prentice Hall, 1983.

Cooper, *Direct Vocal Rehabilitation, Approaches to Vocal Rehabilitation,* Charles C Thomas, 1977.

Crerar, M A & Dean, E C, *Exploring the Potential of Computer Assisted Therapy;* CST Bulletin, October 1984.

Crystal, D, *Prosodic Systems and Intonation in English;* Cambridge University Press, 1969.

Darley, F L, Aronson, A E, & Brown, J R, *Motor Speech Disorders;* W B Saunders & Co., 1975.

Darwin, C J, *On the dynamic use of prosody in speech perception,* 1975, cited in *Clinical Management of Neurogenic Communicative Disorders,* Little, Brown & Co., 1978.

De Jersey, M C, 'An approach to the problems of orofacial dysfunction in the adult'; *The Australian Journal of Physiotherapy,* Volume XXI, 1, 1975.

Dobie, R, 'Rehabilitation of Swallowing Disorders'; *American Family Physician* 17, 5, 84–95, 1975.

DHSS, *Aids for the Disabled:* Leaflet HB2.

Easton, J & Enderby, P, *The Acquisition of Aids for the Speech Impaired,* Frenchay Hospital, Bristol BS16 1LE.

Edwards, M, *Disorders of Articulation;* Springer-Verlag, 1984.

Enderby, P, 'Assisting the patient who has difficulty swallowing'; *College of Speech Therapists Bulletin* No. 388, 1–3. August 1984.

Enderby, P M, *Frenchay Dysarthria Assessment;* College-Hill Press, 1983.

Fawcus, M, Robinson, M, Williams, J & Williams, R, *Working with Dysphasics;* Winslow Press, 1983.

Gordon, M T, Morton, F M & Simpson, I C, 'Airflow measurements in diagnosis, assessment and treatment of mechanical dysphonia'; *Folia Phoniatrica,* 30, 372–379, 1978.

Greene, M C L, *The Voice and its Disorders;* 4th edition, Pitman Medical Publication, 1980.

Grunwell, P & Huskins, S, 'Intelligibility in acquired dysarthria—a neuro-phonetic approach: three case studies'; *Journal of Communicative Disorders,* 12, 9–22, 1979.

Hawkridge, D, Vincent, T & Hales, G, *New Information Technology in the Education of Disabled Children and Adults;* Croom Helm, 1985.

Helm, N A, 'Management of palilalia with a pacing board'; *Journal of Speech and Hearing Disorders,* 44, 350–353, 1979.

Jacobson, E, *You Must Relax,* McGraw-Hill Book Co., 1957.

Kabat, H & Knott, M, 'Proprioceptive facilitation techniques for treatment of paralysis'; *Physical Therapy Review,* 33, 2, 1953.

Knott, M & Voss, D, 'Patterns of motion for proprioceptive neuro-muscular facilitation.' *British Journal of Physical Medicine,* 17, 9, 1954.

Langley, J & Darvill, G, *P.N.F.—A practical manual;* 1979.

Logemann, J, *Evaluation and Treatment of Swallowing Disorders;* College-Hill Press, 1983.

Luria, A R, *Traumatic aphasia: its syndromes, psychology and treatment;* Mouton, 1970.

McNeil, M R, Rosenbek, J C & Aronson, A E, *The Dysarthrias—Physiology, Acoustics, Perception, Management;* College-Hill Press, 1984.

Moncur, J P & Brackett, I P, *Modifying Vocal Behaviour,* Harper and Row, 1974.

Netsell, R, *Normal Aspects of Speech, Hearing and Language;* Prentice-Hall, 1973.

Perkins, M R, 'Application of Computers in Speech Therapy'; *CST Bulletin,* June 1985.

Perkins, W H (ed.), *Dysarthria and Apraxia—Current Therapy of Communication Disorders;* Thieme-Stratton Inc., 1983.

Robertson, S J, *Dysarthria profile;* S J Robertson, Manchester Polytechnic, 1982.

Robertson, S J, 'Dysarthria profile: background and development'; *College of Speech Therapists' Bulletin,* 359, 3, 1982.

Robertson, S J & Thomson, F, 'Speech therapy and Parkinson's disease'; *College of Speech Therapists' Bulletin,* 370, 10–12, 1983.

Robertson, S J & Thomson, F, 'Speech therapy in Parkinson's disease: a study of the efficacy and long term effects of intensive treatment'; *British Journal of Disorders of Communication,* 19, 213–224, 1984.

Rosenbek, J C & La Pointe, L L, *The dysarthrias: Description, Diagnosis and Treatment,* cited in *Clinical Management of Neurogenic Communicative Disorders,* ed. D F Johns; Little, Brown & Co, 1978.

Rowe, G B, 'Treatment of facial paralysis by neuromuscular facilitation techniques'; *The Australian Journal of Physiotherapy,* Vol XXI, 1, 1975.

RICA (Research Institute for Consumer Affairs), *(i) Communication Aids (guide); (ii) Aids for People with Disabilities;* RICA, 14 Buckingham Street, London WC2.

Schiefelbusch, R L (ed.), *Nonspeech Language and Communication: Analysis and Intervention,* University Park Press, 1980.

Schwartz, A H (ed.), *Handbook of Microcomputer Applications in Communication Disorders;* College-Hill Press, 1984.

Scott, S & Caird, F I, 'Speech therapy for patients with Parkinson's disease'; *British Medical Journal,* 24 October, 1981, 283, 1088.

Scott, S, Caird, F I & Williams, B O, *Communication in Parkinson's Disease;* Croom Helm, 1985.

Shaughnessy, A L, Netsell, R & Farrage, J, 'Treatment of a four-year-old with a palatal lift prosthesis'; in *Clinical Dysarthria,* Edited by W R Berry. College-Hill Press, 1983.

Silverman, F H, *Communication for the Speechless;* Prentice-Hall, 1980.

Thomson, F, The use of sign language and the Makaton Vocabulary with adults with acquired speech and language disorders; *College of Speech Therapists' Bulletin,* 361, 1, 1982.

Tonkovich, J D, Latham, T J, & Rambow, M W, *Dysarthria Rehabilitation Programme;* CC Publications/Taskmaster Ltd.

Yorkston, K M & Beukelman, D R, *Assessment of Intelligibility of Dysarthric Speech;* CC Publications Inc/Taskmaster, 1981.

Yorkston, K M & Beukelman, D R, 'Ataxic dysarthria: treatment sequences based on intelligibility and prosodic considerations'; *Journal of Speech and*

DYSARTHRIA SOURCEBOOK

Sandra Robertson, Barbara Tanner & Fay Young (Thomson)

Following the publication of *Working with Dysarthrics* many therapists requested an extension to the practical exercises described in this book. This is therefore the basis on which the *Dysarthria Sourcebook* has been developed.

It is comprised of exercises in the areas of: Articulation; Intelligibility, Stress & Intonation. It provides the therapist with literally hundreds of examples to practise with their patients.

This large format book is wire bound and has been freed of all copyright restrictions so that therapists can easily photocopy the exercises for patients to take home. Clear, large and bold type, combined with the careful page design, makes this manual superb for direct use by your clients.

Approx 200 pages, wire bound, A4.

ISBN 0 86388 071 1